University-Linked Retirement Communities: Student Visions of Eldercare

Leon A. Pastalan
Benyamin Schwarz
Editors

The Haworth Press, Inc.
New York · London · Norwood (Australia)

University-Linked Retirement Communities: Student Visions of Eldercare has also been published as *Journal of Housing for the Elderly,* Volume 11, Number 1 1994.

The development, preparation, and publication of this work has been undertaken with great care. However, the publisher, employees, editors, and agents of The Haworth Press and all imprints of The Haworth Press, Inc., including The Haworth Medical Press and Pharmaceutical Products Press, are not responsible for any errors contained herein or for consequences that may ensue from use of materials or information contained in this work. Opinions expressed by the author(s) are not necessarily those of The Haworth Press, Inc.

The Haworth Press, Inc., 10 Alice Street, Binghamton, NY 13904-1580 USA

Library of Congress Cataloging-in-Publication Data

University-linked retirement communities: student visions of eldercare / Leon A. Pastalan, Benyamin Schwarz, editors.
    p. cm.
    Originally published as v. 11, no. 1 of the Journal of housing for the elderly.
    Includes bibliographical references.
    ISBN 1-56024-570-0 (alk. paper)
    1. Retirement communities–United States. 2. Community and college–United States. 3. University of Michigan–Public services. I. Pastalan, Leon A., 1930–　. II. Schwarz, Benyamin.
HQ1063.2.U6U56 1993
378.1'03–dc20   93-40379
                                                                      CIP

University-Linked Retirement Communities: Student Visions of Eldercare

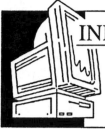# INDEXING & ABSTRACTING

Contributions to this publication are selectively indexed or abstracted in print, electronic, online, or CD-ROM version(s) of the reference tools and information services listed below. This list is current as of the copyright date of this publication. See the end of this section for additional notes.

- *Abstracts in Social Gerontology: Current Literature on Aging*, National Council on the Aging, Library, 409 Third Street, SW, 2nd Floor, Washington, DC 20024

- *Ageline Database*, American Association of Retired Persons, 601 E Street NW, Washington, DC 20049

- *AGRICOLA Database*, National Agricultural Library, 10301 Baltimore Boulevard, Room 002, Beltsville, MD 20705

- *Applied Social Sciences Index & Abstracts (ASSIA) (Online: ASSI via Data-Star) (CD Rom: ASSIA Plus)*, Bowker-Saur Limited, Maypole House, Maypole Road, East Grinstead, West Sussex RH19 1HH, England

- *Architectural Periodicals Index*, The British Architectural Library, RIBA, 66 Portland Place, London W1N 4AD, England

- *Communication Abstracts*, Temple University, 303 Annenberg Hall, Philadelphia, PA 19122

- *GEO Abstracts (GEO Abstracts/GEOBASE)*, Elsevier/GEO Abstracts, Regency House, 34 Duke Street, Norwich NR3 3AP, England

(continued)

- *Human Resources Abstracts (HRA)*, Sage Publications, Inc., 2455 Teller Road, Newbury Park, CA 91320

- *Inventory of Marriage and Family Literature (online and hard copy)*, National Council on Family Relations, 3989 Central Avenue NE, Suite 550, Minneapolis, MN 55421

- *Mental Health Abstracts (online through DIALOG)*, IFI/Plenum Data Company, 3202 Kirkwood Highway, Wilmington, DE 19808

- *OT Bibsys*, American Occupational Therapy Foundation, P.O. Box 1725, Rockville, MD 20849-1725

- *Psychological Abstracts (PsycINFO)*, American Psychological Association, P.O. Box 91600, Washington, DC 20090-1600

- *Public Affairs Information Bulletin (PAIS)*, Public Affairs Information Service, Inc., 521 West 43rd Street, New York, NY 10036-4396

- *Sage Urban Studies Abstracts (SUSA)*, Sage Publications, Inc., 2455 Teller Road, Newbury Park, CA 91320

- *Social Planning/Policy & Development Abstracts (SOPODA)*, Sociological Abstracts, Inc., P.O. Box 22206, San Diego, CA 92192-0206

- *Sociological Abstracts (SA)*, Sociological Abstracts, Inc., P.O. Box 22206, San Diego, CA 92192-0206

- *Urban Affairs Abstracts*, National League of Cities, 1301 Pennsylvania Avenue NW, Washington, DC 20004

(continued)

SPECIAL BIBLIOGRAPHIC NOTES

related to special journal issues (separates) and indexing/abstracting

☐ indexing/abstracting services in this list will also cover material in the "separate" that is co-published simultaneously with Haworth's special thematic journal issue or DocuSerial. Indexing/abstracting usually covers material at the article/chapter level.

☐ monographic co-editions are intended for either non-subscribers or libraries which intend to purchase a second copy for their circulating collections.

☐ monographic co-editions are reported to all jobbers/wholesalers/approval plans. The source journal is listed as the "series" to assist the prevention of duplicate purchasing in the same manner utilized for books-in-series.

☐ to facilitate user/access services all indexing/abstracting services are encouraged to utilize the co-indexing entry note indicated at the bottom of the first page of each article/chapter/contribution.

☐ this is intended to assist a library user of any reference tool (whether print, electronic, online, or CD-ROM) to locate the monographic version if the library has purchased this version but not a subscription to the source journal.

☐ individual articles/chapters in any Haworth publication are also available through the Haworth Document Delivery Services (HDDS).

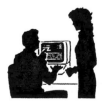

University-Linked Retirement Communities: Student Visions of Eldercare

CONTENTS

PART TWO: STUDENT DESIGN PRESENTATIONS

AFTERWORD

ABOUT THE EDITORS

Leon A. Pastalan, PhD, is Professor of Architecture in the College of Architecture and Urban Planning at the University of Michigan. Dr. Pastalan is also Director of the National Center on Housing and Living Arrangements for Older Americans. As a researcher of long standing in the field of environments for the elderly, he is an expert in sensory deficits, spatial behavior, and housing. Dr. Pastalan has published many books and articles resulting from his work, including *Man Environment Reference 2 (MER 2)*, (The University of Michigan Press, 1983), *Retirement Communities: An American Original* (The Haworth Press, Inc., 1984), *Lifestyles and Housing of Older Adults: The Florida Experience* (The Haworth Press, Inc., 1989), *Aging in Place: The Role of Housing and Social Supports* (The Haworth Press, Inc., 1990), and *Optimizing Housing for the Elderly: Homes Not Houses* (The Haworth Press, Inc., 1991). Dr. Pastalan is also Editor of the *Journal of Housing for the Elderly* (The Haworth Press, Inc.).

Benyamin Schwarz, PhD, is Assistant Professor in the Environmental Design Department at the University of Missouri-Columbia, and Research Associate with the Environmental Design for Aging Research Group at the University of Michigan. Dr. Schwarz has practiced architecture in Israel for several years with a special focus on settings for aging populations. He taught in The College of Architecture and Urban Planning in the University of Michigan and in Eastern Michigan University. His research has addressed the design process of extended care facilities and dementia special care units in the U.S. and abroad.

Introduction:
Elders' Utopia

Designing environments that meet the needs of older populations
is becoming a significant issue in the field of architecture. Like
other fields of inquiry, architects became keenly aware that in the
coming decades the world will experience a dramatic increase in the
number of older people. Recent figures for the United States (U.S.
Senate, 1991) indicate that there are 31.2 million older adults
(12.6% of the population). This number is anticipated to increase to
66 million older persons by the year 2030 (21.8% of the population). The most dramatic increases are occurring in the population
of people 85 years and older, who by the year 2040 will number
approximately 12.25 million (Spencer, 1989). In a White Paper,
published in August 1991 by the American Institute of Architecture
(AIA), the authors argued that in order to meet the design goals of
facilities for aging Americans, education and training needs have to
be extended to architecture students, faculty, researchers, practitio-
ners and their allied professionals and to the entire community
responsible for the built environment for elderly people.

This book grew out of a two-term graduate course offered in the
College of Architecture and Urban Planning at the University of
Michigan during the academic year of 1991-92. The course, which
dealt with aging and environment, focused on theoretical and practical design aspects of a retirement community as an integral part of
a university setting. Structured as a seminar, the first term was
driven by two objectives: (1) to increase students' knowledge in the

[Haworth co-indexing entry note]: "Introduction: Elders' Utopia." Pastalan, Leon A., and Benya-
min Schwarz. Co-published simultaneously in *Journal of Housing for the Elderly* (The Haworth Press,
Inc.) Vol. 11, No. 1, 1994, pp. 1-10; and: *University-Linked Retirement Communities: Student Visions of
Eldercare* (ed: Leon A. Pastalan, and Benyamin Schwarz) The Haworth Press, Inc., 1994, pp. 1-10.
Multiple copies of this article/chapter may be purchased from The Haworth Document Delivery Center
[1-800-3-HAWORTH; 9:00 a.m. - 5:00 p.m. (EST)].

1

area of person-environment interactions through better understanding of behavioral systems of older people; and (2) to examine environmental attributes which constitute an appropriate environment for the elderly. This population is more sensitive to the physical environment due to the inevitable changes in sensory acuity, psychomotor speed, mobility, and social roles. Based on this mission, the students studied issues such as spatial behavior, privacy, personal space, territoriality, wayfinding, person-environment fit, gerontological design problems, barrier-free design, the retirement community phenomenon, long-term care environments, different forms of housing for the elderly, site development patterns, and detailing of facilities for aging populations. As the class unfolded, they had met with developers, retired faculty from the university, and people from the Center for Independent Living. They also did a post-occupancy evaluation of a local retirement community. Each student in the class had to complete seven short assignments and to write a term paper focused on a subject he or she wanted to learn about. In the winter term of 1992 the course took the form of a design studio. Students were asked to design a utopian continuing care retirement community linked to the University of Michigan.

RETIREMENT COMMUNITIES

Planned retirement communities have, over the past twenty-five years or so, established themselves in the United States as a viable housing option for older people. Increasingly older Americans are able financially and otherwise to demand that the market respond to their needs. Many elderly are demanding to have their very particular housing preferences satisfied by highly specialized packages of housing and services.

Retirement communities in response to these demands have been created by a wide diversity of sponsors including religious groups, voluntary associations, real estate developers and others. Many of these entities have developed an isolated, self-sustaining community life while others depend in part or in whole on the service of an outside source. Each type of community involves certain gains and losses with respect to personal and financial security, responsibility, flexibility, privacy and the like.

A national study completed in the early 1980s (Hunt et al. 1984) had shown there were nearly 2,400 retirement communities identified which had a total population of nearly 1,000,000. The communities identified reflected five different types of retirement communities consisting of Retirement New Towns; Retirement Villages; Retirement Sub-divisions; Retirement Residences and Continuing Care Retirement Communities.

Each of these different communities represented a different focus. For instance, New Towns such as Sun City with a population of approximately 50,000 were originally built for healthy, middle and upper-income couples who want a leisurely, but active lifestyle. Retirement Villages are smaller, typically less than 5,000 residents, and they are less self-contained, built for a similar population as Retirement New Towns. Retirement Sub-divisions are communities for the less affluent that take advantage of supportive services in surrounding communities and seldom have more than 500 people.

Retirement Residences typically have non-profit sponsors and house an older, widowed or single population with modest incomes and on average have fewer than 500 people. Continuing Care Retirement Communities (CCRCs) offer a continuum of choices from independent living to nursing care.

Currently there are about 700 planned CCRCs in the U.S. These communities provide housing and health care services to approximately 230,000 residents, most of them over age 75. AAHA and Ernst and Young (1989) defined CCRC as:

> An organization that offers a full range of housing, residential services and health care in order to serve its older residents as their needs change over time. This continuum consists of housing where residents live independently and receive certain residential services such as meals, activities, housekeeping, and maintenance; support services for disabled residents who require assistance with activities of daily living; and health care services for those who become temporarily ill or who require long-term care.

Based on the concept of self-insurance, every continuing care arrangement involves a contract between residents and the CCRC that, at a minimum, guarantees shelter and access to various health care services for the balance of the resident's lifetime. In return the resident agrees to pay a lump-sum entrance fee upon moving to the community and monthly payments thereafter. Most CCRC contracts contain a clause governing refund of the entrance fee if the contract is terminated by the resident and/or if the resident dies. Depending on the contract, entrance fees may be non-refundable, refundable on a declining basis over time, partially refundable, or fully refundable.

Continuing care retirement communities have been in existence for about 100 years. They evolved from the life care communities started by religious and fraternal organizations. Those groups cared for their aged members in return for all their worldly possessions (Consumer Report, 1990). The big expansion of CCRCs started in the 1960s as a response to the major demographic and socioeconomic changes. These include the dramatic growth of the number of elderly in the population, decline of the traditional family homestead, and liberalized pension systems which have lead to greater financial independence for most older people (Somers and Spears, 1992). Most CCRCs are sponsored by religious or other non-profit organizations. While there are many variations, the typical CCRC today averages about 200 independent living apartments, 40 personal care or assisted living beds and 90 skilled nursing beds. The common problems of older people, such as lack of health insurance, difficulty maintaining a home, isolation, lack of activity, increasing frailty, poor nutrition, lack of services, lack of transportation, can almost all be solved or managed within a CCRC. A life care community, as the CCRC is sometimes called, is an approach that appears, at this time, to offer one of the best opportunities for a secure, comfortable, active, and health-care protected future for American elderly (Chellis and Grayson, 1990).

Retirement Communities and Universities

While most planned communities have done a reasonable job of providing for the needs of the body, such as comfortable surroundings, excellent food and good health care, there is relatively little done in the way of sustenance for the soul. By that is meant an environment to enhance independence, personal growth, meaningful work substitutes and companionship of peers. There is a new response emerging that may help satisfy these "finer human hungers." The response is that of a college or university based retirement community. Such a milieu can provide a rich and varied context for older people to be exposed to new ideas and learning, for personal growth and to discover new approaches to a meaningful life. This environment may also serve to reduce the stereotypes and attitudes which the young and old have of each other and in the process enhance the possibilities for interacting and learning across the generations.

PLAN AND FOCUS OF THE BOOK

Three kinds of audiences may benefit from this book: (1) potential users of eldercare services such as elderly people and their families, providers of services in retirement communities, retired faculty, staff, alumni and friends of universities; (2) people who are concerned about aging and environment such as designers, architects, policy makers, developers; (3) educators and students of architecture and other fields who are interested in the combination of housing and care options for senior adults.

This book consists of two parts. The first part comprises edited essays by students of this course. Melissa Lucksinger's *Community and the Elderly* discusses the concept of *community* as it is reflected in ideal and real communities and its meaning in retirement communities for the elderly. Paul Ingman's *Person, Place, and View* is a description of a day in the life of an older person and the engagement with the view from his or her personal space. Michael Nicklowitz's and Kwang-Sun Choi's report, *Retirement Community Site Evaluation* evaluated four sites in Ann Arbor for the retirement community. Daniel Koester's *Public Spaces and Common Areas* and Madelyn Wilder's *Housing for a Retirement Community* reviewed the different physical components of the retirement community.

The site evaluation report is one of the reports that were submitted by the students in partial fulfillment of an assignment in the first term. The students were asked to assume that they have been approached by the University Senior Faculty & Staff Housing Association, Inc., that wants to build a retirement community for the university. As experts on behavioral design and service programming for the elderly, the students were asked to consult with the group about what sort of place would be the best site for this purpose. Their evaluation factors included: (1) Accessibility to: shopping, public transportation, religious services, recreation, parking, medical care, personal services (beauty shop, cleaners, etc.); (2) Compatibility with other plans: master plan, regional medical plans, land use and zoning, social-services delivery; (3) Utilities and services: gas, electricity, water, sanitary sewer, storm sewer, trash pickup, sidewalks, crosswalks; (4) Natural features: topography, vegetation; (5) Incompatible surrounding land use: industrial, juvenile, recreation or school, proximity to the university's main campus, vacancies; (6) Vehicular traffic; (7) Expansion potential; (8) Economics: land costs, existing structure demolition, potential for sharing facilities. Although the report presented here recommended the retirement community on site #2, the students preferred site #1 for the final project.

Part two of this book is dedicated to the final design jury of four students' projects. They represent different approaches to the retirement community for the University of Michigan. Typically, retirement communities include apartments and cottages, sheltered apartments connected to a main dining room and other common areas, assisted living apartments, short-term infirmary and long-term nursing care, and services for residents as well as others in the surrounding area. The students were encouraged to choose the *Continuum of Care* for the community. In other words, each student was allowed to develop his or her program and concepts regarding the components of the retirement community and the philosophy of care.

Melissa Lucksinger's project emphasizes mainly the common spaces in the community. She grappled with the physical elements that shelter a community: buildings, streets, open spaces, and so on in an effort to reduce the disadvantages of an age-segregated living environment managed by an intrusive management team. Madelyn Wilder addresses in her proposal the housing component of the community. Her goal was focused on locating attractive housing near a presently existing campus in order to encourage older persons to come to live close to an educational facility so that the latter serves a wider range of clients and thus contributes to the quality of life of older as well as younger persons. Michael Nicklowitz and Kwang-Sun Choi based their design on Maslow's concept of *hierarchy of needs*. Working as a team, they developed a vision of a retirement community which addresses the changing needs of the residents as they age in place. They created an environment that restores an individual's dignity and encourages frivolity, spontaneity, and creative pursuits. In the fourth project, Daniel Koester and Paul Ingman approached the university retirement community with the motto *celebration of life*. Their project focuses its energy on the rhythms and patterns of life, restoring old age to a period of fulfillment, advantage, enchantment and unparalleled freedom.

At the end of the second term the students presented their projects to faculty and visiting professionals. We chose to record the jury and present it in everyday language as it was used in the session in order to capture the meanings in their natural form. The following participants took part in the design jury: Dr. Nathan Levine, AIA from Southfield, Michigan whose firm designed several retirement communities; Daniel Cinelli, AIA, a principal from OWP&P Architects Incorporated in Deerfield, Illinois; Glen Tipton, AIA, a senior vice president of CS&D in Baltimore, Maryland; Leslie Knight, director of the Midwest regional office of the American Association of Homes for the Aging (AAHA); Joseph Hoadly, AIA from Hobbs & Black Associates in Ann Arbor, Michigan; Helen Naimark, MSW, who administrated the Jewish Federation Apartments in Metropolitan Detroit for several years; Jay Turner, a retirement communities developer and owner; Robert Forman, director of the Alumni Association of The University of Michigan; Assistant Professor Ron Sekulski from the School of Art; Professor Kurt Brandle and Associate Professor Tom Hille from the College of Architecture and Urban Planning, The University of Michigan.

DESIGN STUDIO AND DESIGN JURY

Students of architecture spend much of their time working on tasks that are supposed to be analogues of the tasks which they will encounter in practice. The studio is the heart of architectural education. One third to one half of the required educational program takes place in the design studio. This system is almost two hundred and fifty years old. It has its origins in the French Academy in the early eighteenth century. Each studio varies with the teacher, the school, and the students, but the fundamental structure is relatively fixed: the instructor poses a problem and then works individually with the students as they develop their solutions. At the end of the term the students have to face the design jury. This is still the predominant method used to evaluate students' performance in a design studio. Although they may be called *reviews* or *critiques*, with few exceptions the format of the design jury is virtually the same in every school of architecture. Students orally present their completed design work one by one in front of a group of faculty, visiting professionals, and their classmates. The design jury evaluates the students' work on the spot and publicly critiques each project while the students are expected to defend their work.

Wade (1977) noted that design students learn their profession in the same way that some people have supposedly learned to swim—by being thrown into the water. The student learns "what architecture is about. He is initiated into the architectural profession. He learns what questions the profession is willing to address and what questions it is willing to answer." However, there is a fundamental difference between studio problems and practice problems. First the intended consequences in each context are distinct. In an academic context assignments are composed for didactic reasons where complex problems are simplified and variables are isolated for study. The second difference is that school problems are selected by teachers that elect to deal with the issues they consider most significant. This is why a studio problem can be obscure and conceptual in a way that the problems of practice never are (Cuff, 1991). The third difference concerns the influence of time on design solutions. The design of a major project such as a retirement community may require months or even years of effort by the architect alone, as well as the client's representatives and consultants who make substantial contributions. These figures contrast with the period of fifteen weeks that are commonly allowed for the studio design problem. In spite of these and other serious differences, the studio instruction still remains central to the architectural education system in default of anything better.

APPLYING RESEARCH TO DESIGN

As teachers of architecture we have been concerned about the fact that what students do *not* learn is to test their ideas against the increasingly varied, complex information provided by the scientific disciplines. Furthermore, architecture students are not typically trained to reflect on the people who are imagined to occupy the buildings conceived and designed by them. We believe that the business of architecture is that of "person-environment relations." This course was initiated based on the premise that knowledge of the basic principles of human behavior helps us clarify our understanding of the relationship between environment and behavior. This, in turn, helps architects consider how the environment affords people of different backgrounds and capabilities different aesthetic experiences and activity patterns. Consequently, we made an effort to create in this course a knowledge base, grounded in the realities and the current research in the field of environment and aging.

There are signs that the design process for producing new environments for older people is being slowly affected by environmental research. However, it appears that our society still has no conception of the environmental wholeness when we address aging. Clearly, growing old involves both puzzles and mysteries. Aging and environment is an unusually broad and multidisciplinary field of study. Principally we have not yet been able to structure a satisfying environment for continued aging where the occupants and users are the first cause around which the whole architecture process revolves. The challenge has been analogous to the effort to realize utopia.

The students named the project *Elders' Utopia*. Students of architecture are often allowed to dream. They can create their own utopias without the limiting constraints of reality. Still, utopias have their boundaries. They are not just any dream of impossible perfection. They are ways of looking at situations that have their own history and character. Utopia describes a state of impossible perfection which nevertheless is in some genuine sense not beyond the reach of humanity. This, perhaps, was the essence of this course. Students in this class attempted to define the tradition that set the limits to what utopian environments for aging can do. Nevertheless, they confronted reality not with a measured assessment of the possibilities of change, but with the demand for change. This is the way the world should be. It refuses to accept current definitions of the possible because it knows these to be part of the reality that it seeks to change. Architects have to be able to design better environments for aging which assert the rights and freedoms of elderly people to achieve a more fulfilling life.

Leon A. Pastalan
Benyamin Schwarz
Editors

REFERENCES

American Association of Homes for the Aging, and Ernst and Young. (1989). *Continuing care retirement communities: An industry in action: Analysis and development trends 1989.* Washington, DC: The Association.

Chellis, R. D., and Grayson, P. J. (1990). *Life care: A long-term solution?* Lexington, MA: Lexington Books.

Consumer Reports. (1990). *Communities for the elderly.* (Feb.), 123-131.

Cuff, D. (1991). *Architecture: The story of practice.* Massachusetts Institute of Technology.

Heath, T. (1984). *Method in architecture.* John Wiley & Sons Ltd.

Hunt, M. E., Feldt, A. G., Marans, R. W., Pastalan, L. A., and Vakalo, K. L. (1984). *Retirement Communities: An American Original.* New York: The Haworth Press, Inc.

Somers, A. R., and Spears, N. L. (1992). *The continuing care retirement community: A significant option for long-term care?* New York: Springer Publishing Company.

Spencer, G. (1989). *Projections of the Population of the United States, by Age, Sex and Race: 1988 to 2080.* Washington, DC: Bureau of the Census, Current Population Reports Series P-25, No. 1018.

U.S. Senate Special Committee on Aging and the American Association of Retired Persons. (1991). *Aging America: Trends and Projections.* Washington, DC: USD-HHS Pub. NO (FCoA)91-28001.

Wade, J. (1977). *Architecture, problems and purpose.* New York: Wiley-Interscience.

PART ONE: BACKGROUND PAPERS

Community and the Elderly

Melissa K. Lucksinger

It (housing) seems set up to crowd together unrelated and hermetic nuclear families whose only link with each other is that they have been brought together by some mindless central casting to play bit parts in an incomprehensible urban drama . . . with no attention to providing for community, ever.

–Charles W. Moore, Architect

INTRODUCTION

The majority of species exist in some form of *community.* Most do so instinctively because survival dictates this form of living necessary to existence. Human beings began with tribes, small communities, and/or large extended families; they experienced some form of commitment and desire to unify as a whole. In the begin-

[Haworth co-indexing entry note]: "Community and the Elderly." Lucksinger, Melissa K. Co-published simultaneously in *Journal of Housing for the Elderly* (The Haworth Press, Inc.) Vol. 11, No. 1, 1994, pp. 11-28; and: *University-Linked Retirement Communities: Student Visions of Eldercare* (ed: Leon A. Pastalan, and Benyamin Schwarz) The Haworth Press, Inc., 1994, pp. 11-28. Multiple copies of this article/chapter may be purchased from The Haworth Document Delivery Center [1-800-3-HA-WORTH; 9:00 a.m. - 5:00 p.m. (EST)].

ning, unification was for defense purposes and eventually evolved to psychological needs. While modern life has advanced in most areas from a tribal existence, basic needs of security, stability, dependence and intimacy are being denied by the totally independent society prevalent in America today.

What is community? According to Webster's it is defined as "a group of people residing in the same locality and under the same government . . . having common interests . . . common ownership or participation." The word comes from Latin *communitas,* meaning "fellowship" and *communis,* meaning "common." Modernized ideas of community involve social networks that replace the traditional nuclear family. Daniel Yankelovich writes descriptively about feelings of participation in a community; he states, "Here is where I belong, these are my people, I care for them, they care for me, I am a part of them, they share my concerns. I know this place, I am on familiar ground, I am at home." Yankelovich's reference to home does not mean a physical structure or a financial investment. *Home* implies security and comfort and can affect a person's confidence and relationships with others. With the evolution of modern society and dissolution of the traditional nuclear family, the environment must step forward to help create a sense of home. In examining the environment the necessity for supportive communities emerges. Individual commitment to the community can enhance quality of life by creating social networks that provide for individual support. Although American society was founded on individual freedom, the need for community to elicit loneliness and create a sense of self-worth is urgent in today's society.

UTOPIAN IDEALS

In *Utopia* commitment rather than coercion is the link which creates a self-chosen cooperative that operates according to a higher order of spiritual and natural laws. These laws assume that harmony and cooperation rather than conflict and exploitation are inherent human qualities. In Utopia individual and group interests are congruent ensuing mutual responsibility and trust. In essence, Utopia is "the imaginary society in which humankind's deepest yearnings, noblest dreams, and highest aspirations come to fulfillment, where all physical, social, and spiritual forces work together, in harmony, to permit the attainment of everything people find desirable and necessary"(Kanter, p. 7). Critics claim Utopian plans are an escape from reality, however, they are also new creations; they reject the established order and the generally accepted norms of society in an attempt to achieve the perfect human existence.

The realization of Utopia has often been attempted through the organization of *communes*. Communes are typically value-based, communal societies. The vision, as suggested by the word itself, is of community. There is a voluntary conformity based on commitment of the individual to the collective whole. Through group solidarity the commune exists to serve its members, simultaneously implementing a set of values focused towards the attainment of certain ideals. American communes can be categorized as religious, psychological, or political entities. While differing in their ideological basis they present a variety of common values:

- rejection of established order as sinful, unjust, or unhealthy
- rejection of isolation and alienation
- the possibility of perfection through a restructuring of society
- a recreation of lost unity
- immediacy of actions to attain a goal.

The result in trying to achieve these harmonies has been the attempt at the Utopian community or commune.

An example of one such commune is the Oneida, Community of the Past. The members of this commune referred to themselves as the Kingdom of God on earth. Founder John Humphrey Noyes' vision of Utopia became embodied in the Oneida community which was organized around principles of the primitive Christian church: "The believers possessed one heart and one soul and had all things in common" (Kanter, p. 16). As a religious based community Oneida embodied many of the common values discussed previously. In joining together to achieve these values they followed in the belief that an active sense of participation leads to success and harmony for the whole. Everything, material and spiritual, was shared with the community and in return the community supported the individual. Economic communism and communal living, to the point of complex marriage (free love), informed all aspects of group life.

Family life was replaced by group life; while there was contact between biological parents and children it was kept to a minimum to discourage any kind of "special love." Many parent-child relationships existed between unrelated children, and adults. To ensure "community spirit" and to fight egoism and selfishness they used public criticism. Oneida, as well as many other Utopian communities, was scorned and eventually dissolved due to their deviant behavior, which the outside world viewed as unacceptable. While the Oneida community represents a radical Utopian commune, they did satisfy their basic human needs of community. They banded together to achieve a "better, purer, and more moral life, which the rest of society would eventually adopt" (Kanter, p. 18).

Using the Oneida community as an example, the organization of social order within the Utopian commune often used undesirable means to attain social unity. Through the provision of spiritual and material needs, inherent destructive qualities such as competition and egotism are eliminated. While this is true to the vision of a Utopian community, maintaining total communal commitment often requires means beyond harmony, brotherhood, and peace. For example, in the Oneida community a young boy was reprimanded for showing special love for his mother. In punishment he was forbidden to see his mother for a week. While this is one type of social control, another is described as *mutual criticism*. This involved the individual periodically subjecting himself to a committee for criticism. The subject was to acknowledge criticism in silence and to confess to it in writing; after the experience an individual was 'cleansed' and was considered a better member of society. Although the members seemed to find these methods effective, they are a form of coercion to force conformity to social unity. These tactics reinforce the fact that there has to be some form of social control to create a 'harmonious' community.

As pointed out, the idealized community of the Utopian vision is often hard to implement. In fact, few communes have been able to stand the test of time. Setting logistic and economic problems aside, the main ingredient in communes, commitment, is extremely difficult to maintain. The members work for the community to survive and in return must achieve satisfaction through long-term involvement. Satisfaction and commitment to community can create safety, security, stable group relationships, and high levels of self-esteem and pride. A successful commune must have strong feelings of participation, a heightened sense of belonging to a group. The problem which arises is that group pressure and intense social control exist at an expense to the individual. Organizational problems arise that address this issue:

- how to maintain community without coercion
- how to make decisions to the collective satisfaction
- how to build relationships without exclusiveness
- how to create communal life with autonomy.

There is not an all-inclusive answer to these problems. A focus on the need for reciprocal relationships may be helpful; however, as the Utopian communes have discovered, the need for commitment, especially in deviant groups, is stronger than in general society. As George Simmel described, "The secret society claims the whole individual to a greater extent, connects its members in more of their totality, and mutually obligates them more closely than does an open society of identical content" (Kanter, p. 65). Members of Utopian communes have strived to overcome loneliness through shared dreams and to create meaningful life through a community goal. Their trials, tribulations and successes can serve as models for those trying to build community environments in today's society.

KIBBUTZ

Mirroring the attempts of Utopian communes to create the ideal society of the future, the Israeli Kibbutz created a social system that can be quite advantageous. Martin Buber in 1958 called the kibbutz "an experiment that did not fail" (Rabin, p. 5). As an intentional community the kibbutz extends over 80 years. There are particular economic and social events that created an opening for this type of society. The large Jewish population evacuating Russia and the colonizing of Palestine in the years preceding the State of Israel provided the need for communal living. In settling the barren desert, young idealistic individuals knew that a collective settlement rather than traditional family homesteading was necessary for survival.

Kibbutz life is based on total equality; the ultimate in egalitarian idealism. A homogeneous background made this more plausible, as well as their commitment to the 'perfectibility' of the human being. They sought to return to nature and rear a new type of being who would be less selfish, more secure, and more generous. In working towards these goals they have used the Marxist philosophy that people contribute according to their ability and consume according to their needs. There have been many benefits and downfalls of the system. For example, the establishment of a 'total society'. The totality occurs because it is the kibbutz's responsibility to provide for all the needs of the individual. In return the individual must commit to total participation. This combines two major functions of a social organization into one socioeconomic function. Is this positive or negative? It may be argued to either point; however, it is a solution to the need for commitment. Without the usual social and economic divisions that fragment a society the kibbutz stands a greater chance of maintaining commitment from its members. Analyzing on a cost benefit basis, if the quality of life in the kibbutz produces satisfaction for its members, they will work to maintain this standard. However, if the kibbutz members feel they have been 'wronged' the commitment to a total society will be severed.

Many studies have been conducted on the impact of living communally. In a study by Rabin and Hallahmi they presented data collected on the differences between being raised in the kibbutz society and the moshav (traditional Israeli settlement) nuclear family. While they were hesitant to make sweeping generalizations on the impact of a communal environment, they did find that it affected individual life. The kibbutz group demonstrated higher levels of self-actualization as a life-goal, lower levels of friendship intimacy, and viewed their parents more critically than the traditionally socialized group. However, there were many areas in which they found no differences, such as marital status, contribution to society as a life goal, present attachment to parents, and self-esteem. Once again these data can be interpreted in various ways, but some basic facts exist. The lack of extensive immediate family contact does not cause a deficiency in attachment and the continuity of the overall structure aids socialization in the kibbutz.

The kibbutz has a variety of failures and successes in its way of life just as other forms of society. Viewing the kibbutz's positive aspects, society today could learn a great deal about the benefits of communal living. Sociologist Robert Bellah suggests "that our individualism has become unbalanced, creating a culture of separation which, if left unchecked, will collapse of its own incoherence" (McCammant and Durett, p. 196). To remedy the growing isolation and loneliness in our culture today, a look to the kibbutz for a renewed sense of commitment to the community can help guide the efforts that are necessary.

COHOUSING

Changing demographics are occurring across society leaving no one untouched. The ideological 'nuclear family' is almost extinct in American society today. While economic changes are striving ahead, social ideals are lagging behind. Factors at one time taken for granted–family, community, and a sense of belonging–are at a severe point of deficiency. Cohousing takes these ideas and redesigns the concept of neighborhood to fit contemporary lifestyles. It combines the autonomy of private dwellings with advantages of community living.

Cohousing attempts to provide environmental support for the creation of a modern family. It developed as a grass roots movement that grew from dissatisfaction with living places that did not accommodate basic needs. In existing neighborhoods socialization was removed from the community and support was not available. Currently in American housing the single-family detached home constitutes 67 percent of housing stock. Less than one-quarter of the United States' population lives in a nuclear family situation. What does all of this mean? To the Cohousing movement it means it is time for change.

Cohousing as an intentional community differs from previous communes in that it is not based on strong ideological beliefs or a charismatic leader. Cohousing promotes no ideology other than the desire for a more practical and social home environment. There are common facilities, such as dining, laundry services, shops, playrooms, etc., and the basis for use of these spaces is voluntary. Approximately once a month two adults and one child assume the responsibility of making dinner for the community, which can range from 40 to 250 people. The main kitchen is designed for this function and those who wish to attend dinner from the community do so. Through community activities like this neighbors learn each others' skills and feel comfortable asking for assistance because they realize in time they will reciprocate.

The *choice* of involvement is a key concept in cohousing. A participatory process is emphasized from the beginning with residents involved in planning, designing, and being responsible for final decisions. The design of the community emphasizes aspects which encourage social contact:

- intentional neighborhood design
- extensive common facilities (in addition to private)
- resident management
- shared facilities with the community at large.

With these elements planned the establishment of a sense of community occurs relatively quickly. Cohousing, based on this sense of community, provides an environment conducive to communal living and focused on support of the individual.

COMMUNITY ARCHITECTURE

The crucial issue today is how to give people more pride in their environment, involvement in their housing and more control over their lives, all this leading to increased confidence and hope, a development of new organizational skills and a consequent flourishing of new enterprise. We are talking about the regeneration of thousands of local communities . . . To restore hope we must have a vision and source of inspiration.

–The Prince of Wales, June 13, 1986

This royal endorsement gave the English movement of *community architecture* the respectability and credibility it needed to propel itself forward in society. The term community architecture encompasses community planning, designing, development, and technical aid (Wates and Knevitt, p. 17). Community architecture creates a direct relationship between the built environment and the user through control and participation. The critical issue involves giving people more pride in their environment, involvement in their housing, and increased control over their lives. Pioneering projects have demonstrated it is possible to:

- build housing that people want to live in
- reinforce pride and identity with the local community
- build social facilities that are necessary and maintained
- develop neighborhoods and cities that are responsive to people's needs.

The lesson learned from these projects is that "the environment works better if the people who live, work and play in it are actively involved in its creation and management" (Wates and Knevitt, p. 18). Citizens have accepted the responsibility of a creative partnership with politicians and bureaucrats for the creation of harmonious communities. A strong commitment to user participation can satisfy fundamental needs for control and lead to the ability to act individually and collectively. They have focused on the current unprecedented change and diversity in society and on discarding dependency, hierarchy and short-term goals to be replaced with goals of self-help, networking, and long term effects.

In the search for a communal existence the British movement has realized that these idealistic goals can be made concrete. Whether a Utopian commune or an approach to housing, participation and pride in the environment can spark the necessary level of commitment and bring increased hope and confidence to the community.

SOCIETAL CHANGES

As stated previously the transformation of society has begun. The challenge now is to support these changes instead of repeatedly denying them. The change in family structure has implications beyond its immediate participants. The elderly as a group have also been affected, consequently losing their status in society. They are no longer viewed as experienced persons with knowledge to share;

instead, they have become a burden that cannot be dealt with. This may be attributed to the fast-paced, stressed lifestyle prevalent in the work force today and its cultish obsession with youth. Rather than relying on experience for decision making, the desire for technological innovation surpasses the reliance on seniors as knowledgeable contributors. Mass media has also contributed to the negative images of the elderly. Popular television shows and 'news' convey elderly people as helpless, creating a pervasive stigma of worthlessness associated with them. Also traced to societal changes is the alteration in the sense of home. Society has become nomadic; the individual or the family will be easily uprooted to chase vague promises. The idea of home as the extended family has become almost extinct because the family is spread from coast to coast and time is too valuable to share with others.

While these changing demographics and societal values appear negative when presented in this manner, the idea is not to redefine society but to provide the elements necessary to accommodate modern life. By providing a sense of identity for the individuals, old or young, they begin to relate better to the community as a whole because they have achieved confidence in themselves. Through the creation of a sense of home, the feeling of belonging is easier to achieve. Once the individuals become comfortable with their place in society they can then begin to give and take from the community as a whole. The community begins to take over some of the support functions of the traditional nuclear family. Often the community can better provide for the individual because the intense emotional attachment of family is not involved. However, this does not suggest that communal society is necessarily better than family; the implications are that communal society has a lot to offer that is not available in the detached single-family neighborhoods prevalent today.

ELDERLY NEED FOR COMMUNITY

The elderly population is able to benefit from communal order in most instances. With the change in status of seniors many are left in isolation. As a ninety-year-old architect and suffragette who has lived for thirty years in a community says: "Living alone is not a human way to live. You come home to a dark house, cook your dinner, eat by yourself. You go to bed by yourself, and you get up by yourself. It's just not a human way to live" (Porcino, p. xxv). Community supports basic needs that are left unaddressed in an individual existence. It accommodates security, can ease financial burdens, and provide emotional stability. While some communities are focused on reducing expenses, others promise lifetime care regardless of the individuals' availability of resources (after an initial fee) to pay for services. As for emotional stability, the basis of modern community has been to provide the building blocks which are not available in society.

Research supports the fact that the more homogeneous the group the easier supports are developed because members are more likely to have similar interests. By taking advantage of a supportive environment the elderly have the time and energy left over to enjoy a sense of place. In attaining this goal the variables involve more psychological factors than tangible factors of the dwelling itself. However, by providing a physical environment in which the ideals of community can flourish, the individual is aided in feelings of self-worth and commitment to the community, therefore, creating a stronger association with the 'place'. The authors of *If I Live to be 100. . .* sum up the phenomenon well with their statement: "It may seem paradoxical to advocate communal living as the best way to achieve independence. . . . The two go very well together, that the support and interaction with an empathetic community of our peers can make us stronger even when we are more frail" (Carlin and Mansbery, p. 130).

COMMUNAL PROBLEMS

While communal life seems to offer a great number of benefits, problems do arise. As in the community models mentioned above, Utopian communes, the kibbutz, cohousing, and community architecture, the key ingredient is choice. The ability to participate if so desired and the ability of the individual to determine the amount of participation can define the availability of choice. This seems to be an idealistic desire, and the realization of this goal can be quite difficult. For a community to exist there has to be participation from its members, but without using methods of coercion. How is it guaranteed that all members will contribute their necessary share? Along those lines, is it acceptable for a member of the community to benefit from others' work without contributing in return? These questions are difficult to generalize because there is not a specific *recipe* for the creation of community. The closest answer may lie in the level of commitment each member devotes to the community. By attaining a high level of commitment the problem of participation is reduced because those who are committed want to contribute to the whole. Then the focus is shifted to producing dedication for commitment based on a reciprocal relationship between the individual and society. It does not have to achieve the total society provided by the kibbutz; however, the community must offer something (not necessarily monetary) to the individual in return for participation.

If people are satisfied with their involvement in the community, they will be more likely to remain committed to communal living and what they consider its benefits. Concurrently, problems of total commitment must also be addressed. Christopher Alexander describes the theory of *capsule syndrome*. He relates the nuclear submarine and the space capsule, which have no possibility of escape, to total environments (Chermayeff and Alexander, p. 46). The completely man-made character of the capsule creates anxiety of confinement and produces unbearable nervous stress. In focusing on communal living it is necessary to sustain a balanced environment that does not create the need for escape. Describing this perfect stable state of existence Alexander states, "It would be a fully functioning framework for ecological equilibrium."

AGING GROUP CONSCIOUSNESS

While communal living does have problems, it may be the answer to the displacement of elderly persons in today's society. The continued graying of America and the unstructured, uprooted family life has increased the amount of elderly people facing their independent roles in society. As seniors begin to lose touch with cherished roles such as: parent, spouse, wage-earner, community pillar, whatever the case may be, that person must readjust and create a new niche.

One theory that defines this need for alternatives is *disengagement*. The basis of this theory is that in preparing for the ultimate 'disengagement' of death, it is natural for the elderly to want to withdraw from social situations and for society to approve of this behavior (Carlin and Mansberg, p. 126). Contrary to this belief many think that society is coercing this process of disengagement, causing destruction to both groups. Researchers have found that to the elderly activity is not the sole determinant of morale. Positive identification with a similar group can be an equal, if not greater, component in life satisfaction.

This idea leads to the necessity to create a subculture to maintain independence without the participation of society as a whole. Subculture is defined as: "a group that develops in response to isolation and negative evaluation by the larger general culture" (Carlin and Mansberg, p. 127). This acceptance rather than denial of aging leads to an aging group consciousness, which can positively address problems of the aged in a constructive manner. The recognition and acceptance of one's aging allows for the formation of peer friendships and acceptance of peer roles; therein, paving the way for the existence of community.

In summation of the data presented the ultimate question is: does the community aid the elderly? There have been many benefits acknowledged, such as:

- prolonging life and forestalling institutionalization
- achievement of a better quality of life
- maximization of social interaction
- creating a new role for the aged
- role status becomes based on community life, not previous experiences
- maintaining positive relations between children and parents.

These advantages point towards the realization that community living for the elderly can create life rather than contribute to its deterioration. The move to communal living should be voluntary and made before bad health makes it mandatory. Success in creating or joining community relies on the congruence of community and individual ideals in areas of freedom, independence and privacy. A variation in the amount of participation and support exists in the housing options available to the elderly in the form of community.

ALTERNATIVE HOUSING

Alternative communities have been formed in industrialized countries around the world. Alternative housing includes types of housing which are non-traditional, in other words, a deviation from "independent, planned, federally assisted housing" (Blackie et al., p. 7). The range is from one-to-one shared housing to large intentional communities. Each has a distinctive flavor and variation in the communal approach:

> *Elderly Cottage Housing Opportunity (ECHO)* attempts to reintegrate seniors with their families based on the Australian model of granny flats, small mobile living units rented and located near the family home (usually in the backyard). Positively, this helps to unite the family and regain some of the values of a nuclear family. However, the negative side emerges in the dependence of the elderly on family members who may not have the time and the loss of availability of communal benefits to the elderly.

> *Accessory Apartments* provide a self-contained apartment within a single family home. The physical privacy of the apartment distinguishes it from shared living. The resulting atmosphere can be positive if the participants are satisfied; however, with limited contact and a small group the sense of community cannot be achieved.

> *Shared Housing* is a situation in which two or more unrelated people live together in a dwelling unit sharing ownership, household expenses, and responsibilities. The sense of participation in management of the house is high and an individual can make a large contribution to the whole because of the limited group size.

Cooperatives are based on group ownership and participation of the members to maintain the project. Interests and rights of the members, as well as duties and responsibilities, are defined, thus fostering a high level of democracy and community spirit.

Intentional Communities like cooperatives involve the elderly living together cooperatively; in addition, their main focus is on common values and common purpose. This bond creates more homogeneous surroundings which foster community; however, they can also promote the need for escape.

Continuing Care Retirement Communities support the idea of Aging in Place. Through the provision of a range in living from individual to skilled nursing care, members join and stay committed to the community for life (ideally). As a form of intentional community the CCRC can provide support necessary to the individual; however, the stigma of "waiting to die" can deteriorate the sense of community.

These living arrangements are presented from the least communally oriented to the most. Ultimately, they provide what is necessary–a choice. Some individual considerations in joining community involve:

- who to live with (physically and ideologically)
- what type of environment (climatic and density)
- amount of services desired
- ability and desirability of group association.

While communal living may not be the answer for everyone it merits consideration. The living arrangements available offer more support than the single-family detached dwelling unit, but there is much room for new developments to inspire, promote, and educate on alternative housing.

A UNIVERSITY MODEL

Opportunities for the elderly to begin community building exist where many people gain their first and only insight into community living, the university. A university has an unique atmosphere for a number of reasons. First, the majority of students are relatively the same age and have a common focus, to attend the university. Within this general framework there is diversity in the specific lifestyles; some people live alone, some share rooms, and others participate in some form of community. Students are given a choice and, therefore, they are willing to participate in what interests them. The result is a multifaceted environment that offers many opportunities to its members.

While students have been the main focus of campus activities, ranging from community building to lecture attending, faculty also has much to gain from and offer to the university beyond traditional teaching. When retirement age is reached it may not be in everyone's best interests to remove experienced faculty from the learning process. Faculty members, whether they are 45-years-old or 65-years-old, have experience that is vital to the survival of a university. To capitalize on this aspect a community for older faculty in association with the university merges the best of both worlds. The faculty are available to the university and can enjoy the setting in which they are content. Faculty members have a unique common bond in that they obviously enjoy the university setting, where they have probably spent most of their lives. The homogeneity of the faculty members serves to encourage community building and involvement with society. Simultaneously, the combination of old and young also provides a cross generational socialization process in which many people are not involved.

The opportunity for young people to work with senior citizens and learn more about them outside of the classroom helps society as a whole. As young people learn about the elderly, incorrect stereotypes can be broken down and the barriers society has erected between the young and the elderly will begin to disintegrate. The young are gaining from the old and the old are feeling wanted and needed by society. The opportunities in this type of arrangement are countless. Community building is encouraged due to the homogeneous group, the university atmosphere supports diversity and continuity, and the continual learning process of life is that much more enriched.

FUTURE INNOVATIONS

With the realization of the major consequences of modernization in developed societies, an aging population presents major challenges. Care of the elderly has traditionally been the responsibility of the family. However, supports other than that of the nuclear family are required. The previous 'quick fix' bureaucratic programs that can be standardized and delivered to the elderly in the form of shelter and services are ineffective in providing for supportive environments. The issues turn to what is appropriate and desirable, not to the creation of immediate solutions.

The trend is away from historical institutional models of living for the elderly. Through the increase in research and heightened community awareness, necessary options for the elderly are becoming more evident. The need for a 'home-like' environment is being realized. While elderly persons may not regain their previously respected status in American society, they also cannot be discarded and lumped together under an incorrect stereotype. By discarding this stigma the elderly can begin to retain their independence and participate in their own decision making. The freedom of choice for the elderly, as well as general society, can be acknowledged in communal living. In exercising their autonomy older persons can attain emotional and physical reliance from their surroundings. The transformation of the environment from a rudimentary, primitive tribal existence to a 'modern' individualistic society is indicative of the fact that change is the only constant in society. In manipulating the environment to achieve a humane existence, the appropriate response to change will dictate the success of a community.

BIBLIOGRAPHY

Blackie, Norman et al. *Alternative Housing and Living Arrangements for Independent Living*. Ann Arbor, Michigan: The University of Michigan.

Campanale, Eugene A. "Students and Adults Caring For Each Other," *College Student Journal*, Vol. 18, No. 2. Project Innovation, 1984.

Carlin, Vivian F. and Mansberg, Ruth. *If I Live to Be 100. . . Congregate Housing for Later Life*. West Nyack, New York: Parker Publishing Company, Inc., 1984.

Chermayeff, Derge and Alexander, Christopher. *Community and Privacy Toward a New Architecture of Humanism*. New York, New York: Doubleday and Company, Inc., 1963.

Clark, Margaret and Anderson, Barbara G. *Culture and Aging.* Springfield, Illinois: Charles C Thomas, 1967.

Egerton, John. *Visions of Utopia.* Knoxville, Tennessee: The University of Tennessee Press, 1977.

Kanter, Rosabeth M. *Commitment and Community.* Cambridge, Massachusetts: Harvard University Press, 1972.

Marcus, Clare C. and Sarkissian, Wendy. *Housing as if People Mattered.* Berkeley, California: University of California Press, 1986.

McCammant, Kathryn and Durrett, Charles. *Cohousing A Contemporary Approach to Housing Ourselves.* Berkeley, California: Habitat Press, 1989.

Porcino, Jane. *Living Longer, Living Better.* New York, New York: The Continuum Publishing Company, 1991.

Rabin, A.I and Beit-Hallahmi, Benjamin. *Twenty Years Later Kibbutz Children Grown Up.* New York, New York: Springer Publishing Company, 1982.

Schwartz, Benjamin. Personal Interview. November 1991.

Smithers, Janice A. *Determined Survivors.* New Brunswick, New Jersey: Rutgers University Press, 1985.

Sneddon, Jim and Theobald, Caroline. *Building Communities.* London: Community Architecture Information Services Ltd., 1987.

Streib, Gordon F., Folts, W.E., and Hilker, Mary Anne. *Old Homes-New Families: Shared Living for the Elderly.* New York, New York: Columbia University Press,1984.

Wates, Nick and Knevitt, Charles. Community Architecture. London: Penguin Books, 1987.

Person, Place, and View

Paul Christian Ingman

INTRODUCTION

Design must incorporate the deeper meaning of a view into the daily lives of older people. The fact that elderly people spend more time than others indoors increases the need and importance of a view.

In contrast, design often neglects the positive benefits between a person, place and view. The elderly who are bedridden often confront the restrictions of a medical bed and standard window heights. An immobile person may find themselves in a environment that is dysfunctionally linked to their needs and concerns. Indeed, generic or standardized environments do not serve the diverse visual or cognitive needs of an older person. Generic solutions often emerge as something less than empathic toward the expectations of older people.

Because many experiences are woven into the life of an elderly person, design must incorporate views that contribute to the quality, intensity and meaning of a person's life. Design must enrich the transformation of night into daylight, link to a natural environment, connect to a broader social activity, accent the changing seasons/weather and bring the habitat of the wildlife into concert with an elderly person's life. When common visual experiences are thoughtfully manipulated through design, a view becomes a manifestation of the person's newfound freedom.

[Haworth co-indexing entry note]: "Person, Place, and View." Ingman, Paul Christian. Co-published simultaneously in *Journal of Housing for the Elderly* (The Haworth Press, Inc.) Vol. 11, No. 1, 1994, pp. 29-36; and: *University-Linked Retirement Communities: Student Visions of Eldercare* (ed: Leon A. Pastalan, and Benyamin Schwarz) The Haworth Press, Inc., 1994, pp. 29-36. Multiple copies of this article/chapter may be purchased from The Haworth Document Delivery Center [1-800-3-HA-WORTH; 9:00 a.m. - 5:00 p.m. (EST)].

Every day people's lives are filled with views of places and things that reaffirm who they are in the society. The combination of these views and their meaning over a lifetime contribute to shape a person's visual and cognitive expectations. These expectations can be achieved through design. Designing a view offers an elderly person the opportunity to participate in the social activities of a larger community and the amenities of a natural world. Such visual experiences become places that are able to stimulate the visual curiosity of those who are physically isolated.

This paper presents an imaginary stroll in the life of an elderly person who lives in a full service retirement community. Here design has been thoughtfully linked to the attributes of a spectacular view. The view has been designed to enhance the cognitive expectations of elderly people and their activities of daily living. This paper will identify the design implications that are associated with these views showing that a view offers a variety of visual stimuli for the elderly person through content, light and place. This imaginary story takes place in a second floor apartment that overlooks a major metropolitan city. The apartment looks onto a city park, a panorama view of the city's skyline and to the social activities in the community along the river shore drive. This imaginary story begins at sunrise on a sunny summer day in the life of a single eighty-four year old healthy independent person who is about to awaken.

THE MORNING SUNRISE

Sunlight begins to filter into my bedroom around the edges of the window drapes. The warmth of the early morning sun merges with the expectations of the coming day: When should I get up? What do I have planned? What will the weather be like? The sun's bright and reflective warmth fills the early morning. Out from the darkness the city's landscape reveals itself to me from my bed as the electronically controlled drapes slowly replace the night with the morning's first light. I look for changes that have occurred during the night.

I look beyond the park's river of trees and toward the sunrise and the golden light that reflects off the city of glass. I see the city's rhythm. Neighbors tend their gardens, children play, birds nest, people and cars move to deliver services. I see things of interest that are different from my own private world.

The morning view of the community and its surroundings brings me into harmony with a larger purpose and meaning of life. My view permits me to participate in the community's daily activities and the lives of others, if only visually, no matter how isolated or immobile I may become in the future.

The morning sun penetrates into the innermost reaches of my personal space. The natural light allows me to see, rise from the bed and helps me to find my way to my clothes. I open the closet doors which face the source of the daylight. My closet fills with light and reflects the colors of my clothes throughout the closet space.

I remove my clothes and enter the bathroom. The bathroom offers me daylight and yet privacy. From the watercloset I can see the panoramas of nature's dramatic setting. I am never concerned about my visual privacy because the design has insured that I can see without being seen.

I prepare my morning bath under the spacious full ceiling skylight. The light reflects through the bath water, alters and returns its bluish fluttering shapes throughout my space. I touch the water and carefully check its temperature. Handrails provide support. I enter the bath through the soft glow of the early morning light. I sunbathe and soak in the warm water as I overlook the outdoor view. I immerse myself in the golden light offered by the view from my private world.

I remove the sparkling water from the bath. I dry and groom myself. I manicure my nails because it's easier to perform this task in the daylight. I dress for the activities of the day within my sunlit space.

I enter the kitchen to prepare and eat my breakfast. The kitchen's view is of the railroad station in the distance. The kitchen's stain-glass clearstory reflects its rainbow of colors throughout the space. The natural light in the kitchen is more than ample for me to visually function with knives and utensils. I can easily see by the sunlight to serve myself and eat. After eating I clean the smooth ceramic cook top surfaces that are flush with my counter tops. I turn and wash dishes in the natural light that reflects rainbows through the soapy bubbles. I clean my apartment. I await my guests who will soon arrive. I typically clean my apartment in the morning because my energy level is higher. I have ample natural light to dust and to see cob-webs in the corners of my apartment which are often hard to see under artificial light. I find the morning is always the best time to clean.

I water and care for my interior plants under my greenhouse skylight, which frames the outdoor views and diffuses the direct sunlight. The greenhouse skylight is a source of fresh air and fragrance for my apartment.

THE AFTERNOON

As I prepare lunch for my guests, I can easily see to read the cookbook recipes, search and reach for spices and dishes on the shelves of my sunlit space. I rarely have difficulty seeing under the kitchen's central skylight. The kitchen skylight brings sunlight into the center of the food preparation area. Extra sunlight is provided by the large windows that have been thoughtfully placed along the counters and oriented in such a way as to avoid the unflattering views of some surrounding areas. However, the placement of these windows allows an abundance of indirect sunlight.

My guests arrive and are ushered into the foyer. The foyer is the sunlit hub of my apartment. The foyer offers my guests a softened natural light. This soft natural light is provided through the upper clearstory windows that also gently spill light into the adjacent spaces. The foyer's clearstory imparts a buttery warmth over my guests and escorts us into other spaces within my apartment. We move toward the window place, where we will sit and converse.

Once my guests and I arrive at the window place, we are able to look out at a city and its surrounding park-like scenery. Why do guests always compliment "me" on the spectacular view? My friends choose to relax and spend time comfortably lounging. The window place washes us with warm indirect light from the sun. The sunlight that once drew us to the window place now shows us that the importance of this place is the view. This window commands control over the scenery, the river and the city skyline. These windows allow a view from deep within the space.

The intense sunlight is unable to enter directly through the tinted windows or under the extended overhangs. We remain cool. The design prevents direct sunlight, harsh glares and reflections from streaming into the apartment. The direct sunlight is prevented from entering other spaces because of screens, blinds or opaque glass. The orientation and arrangement of these apartment openings accommodate the climatic features, views and other weather considerations.

We venture outdoors onto the deck, where we sit in the warmth of the sun. From the deck we can admire the mountains in the distance. The sunlit deck is surrounded by my plants and flowers which I grew under my special greenhouse skylight. We sit under the tree canopy that was planned in such a way as to screen less desirable views of office and industrial buildings. The view beyond the trees and near the terrain is where people play with their colorful kites that soar high above the other parklike activities. I feel fortunate to visually participate and share in the experience of others with my guests. These views sustain our interest and foster forgotten memories.

One guest exclaims, "Can you see the squirrel?" The other person said, "Fantastic! They are so acrobatic and athletic it's unbelievable." I said, "How can he do that?" My guest said, "That's a good question. Just think of the body control and also the equilibrium. Those creatures are fearless. They manage to reach out for the last fruits on the branch." Our view of the squirrels and birds, woodchucks and other wildlife provide us delight and entertainment.

As my guests leave they speak of my apartment's sunlight that offered them an airy and spacious apartment. I am fortunate that my apartment is alive and filled with familiar experiences and things from the activities of the life outdoors. I never feel cooped-up or isolated from the activities of outdoors. I visually participate in my community. I welcome the natural environment and the social activities of others to intrude into my private world. I value unrestricted vistas that provide me new experiences. The natural features that surround my apartment continually elicit positive feelings about my place and myself. These views will always foster restorative feelings in my life.

THE EVENING SUNSET

The sunset transforms day into night. The sunset reverses my apartment's privacy into a beacon for the world to see. I manipulate my apartment's environment in an attempt to preserve my autonomy from the city. The sunset from the western sky reflects its colors throughout my apartment's surfaces. The sunset transforms my once common possessions into unfamiliar things that shimmer with colorful light. The sunset's brilliance slowly turns its color into darker shades. This evening the city lights will strive to infuse with my apartment's private world.

Tonight my dinner will be catered. I will be surrounded by the full length interior mirror that will soon echo the city's night lights and its activities throughout the surfaces of my space. The interior windows, glass doors and sidelights will enable the lights from the city of mid-town to be shared by every space within my apartment. The city's evening lights will soon intensify. I will watch the shadowy pedestrian figures that move and jog along the shoreline beneath the amber lights.

Before I go to bed, I sit for the last time by the window. The window place provides me a cozy vantage point to view the evening's activities, to sit or to read. This evening the special place admits a breathtaking and expansive vista. I observe the city turning on its artificial lights. The city's lights filter through the trees as the summer breeze begins to ripple a reflection of the city across the water. I see the methodical movements of vehicles twisting their colored lights through the distant luminous city. This panoramic lens of the city reveals a calmer and quieter nature to the city that prepares to rest.

THE NIGHT TIME

I awaken. I move to the bathroom under the continuous moonlit corridor skylight. The corridor skylight provides me ample moonlight to see without the shock and glare of artificial light. I wash and return to bed through the same filtered moonlight that enters through the skylight. The moonlight guides me through my apartment. The moonlight reflects off the dramatic park landscape beyond my darkened apartment.

I pass the special place in my apartment where the view aligns with a small window slit in the wall. The window slit provides for an instant, intense view of a distinctive landmark. This view is so restrained by design that its view will remain alive forever. The moonlight begins to fade over my once public view. I return to bed. Sleep weaves the special memories of the day into the dark and deep shadows of my private world.

CONCLUSION

This paper has sought to demonstrate that it is unreasonable to treat an elderly person's visual experience as less relevant than the traditional issues associated with an older person's activities of daily living. Older people, if isolated from a view for any length of time, need to be refreshed and to look out at a world that is different from their own. They need to look at a world that is familiar but yet holds the promise of more information.

Designing a view can achieve the cognitive expectations of older people. Such designs offset the daily deprivation associated with decreased visual functioning, reduced mobility and diminished stamina. Consequently, design has a responsibility to avoid imprisonment or detachment of the elderly from a public world but must permit the deeper meaning of life to emerge and to flourish through the triangulation between person, place and view.

BIBLIOGRAPHY

Alexander, Christopher, *A Pattern Language: Towns–Building Construction*, Oxford University Press, New York, 1977.

Biner, Paul, "An Arousal Optimization of Model Lighting Preferences," *Environment and Behavior*, Vol. 21, No. 1, January 1989.

Butler, Darrell, "A Preliminary Study of Skylight Preferences," *Environment and Behavior*, Vol. 22, No. 1, January 1990.

Butler, Darrell, "Effects of Setting on Window Preferences and Factors Associated with those Preferences," *Environment and Behavior*, Vol. 21, No. 1, January 1989.

Campbell, Scott S., "Exposure to Light in Healthy Elderly Subjects and Alzheimer's Patients," *Physiology & Behavior*, Vol. 42, 1988.

Carstens, Diane, "The Aging Process and Designing for the Elderly General Issues," *Site Planning and Design for the Elderly*, Van Nostrand Reinhold, 1985.

Dietsch, Deborah, "Record Houses 1989," *Architectural Record*, Mid-April 1989.

Eifrig, David and Kenneth Simons, "An Overview of Common Geriatric Ophthalmologic Disorders," *Geriatrics*, Vol. 38, No. 4, April 1983.

Gaskie, M., "A Little Help: Housing for the Aging," Architectural Record, April 1988.

Heerwagen, Judith, "Affective Functioning, Light Hunger, and Room Brightness Preferences," *Environment and Behavior*, Vol. 22, No. 1, September 1990.

Kane, Robert, *Essentials of Clinical Geriatrics*, New York: McGraw Hill, 1989.

Kaplan, Rachel, "The Role of Nature on the Urban Context," Altman and Wohlwill, *Behavior and the Natural Environment*, New York: Plenum, 1983.

Keep, P., "Stimulus Deprivation in Windowless Rooms," *Anaesthesia*, 32, 1977.

Lam, William, *Sunlight as Form giver for Architecture*, Van Nostrand Reinhold, 1986.

L., Barbara and P. Whieley, "Bringing in Daylight . . . with a Hall," Sunset, January 1992.

Marcus Copper, Clare and Wendy Sarkissian, *Housing as if People Mattered*, University of California Press, Berkeley, 1986.

Moore-Ede, Martin C., "Circadian Timekeeping in Health and Disease," *The New England Journal of Medicine*, September 1, 1983.

Pastalan, L., "The Empathic Model–Methodological Bridge Between Research and Design."

Ruys, T., "Windowless Offices," Unpublished M. Arch. Thesis, Seattle: University of Washington, 1970.

Sauer, David M., "The Great Wall of Glass," *Qualified Remodeler,* Volume 17, Number 14, December 1991.

Soloman, Daniel, "Glencove Houses, Vallejo," *Architectural Record*, August 1988.

Stern, Robert, "Office for Capital Research Company, New York," *Architectural Record,* Mid-September 1989.

Sussman, Alfred and Selma, Interview by author, 27 November 1991, Ann Arbor, Tape recording by Paul Christian Ingman, College of Architecture and Urban Planning, The University of Michigan.

Takahashi, Joseph and Martin Zatz, "Regulation of Circadian Rhymicity," *Science,* Vol. 217, September 17, 1982.

Theodore, H. Koff, "National Overview of the Elderly Population," *Journal of Architectural Education,* Vol. XXXI (1), September 1977.

Ulrich, Roger, "View Through a Window May Influence Recovery from Survey," *Science*, Vol. 224, April 27, 1984.

Verderber, Stephen, "Windowless and Human Behavior in the Hospital Rehabilitation Environment," (Doctor of Arch. dissertation, University of Michigan, 1983).

Retirement Community Site Evaluation

Michael Nicklowitz
Kwang-Sun Choi

INTRODUCTION

The intent of this study is to compare four individual sites in the city of Ann Arbor for the development of a senior housing project. This proposed housing development will be used by retired faculty and staff of the University of Michigan. This study is to examine the potential and relative amenities each site has to offer in a systematic and comparative evaluation. Due to the variety of lifestyles of seniors in our society, it is impossible to say that any one site is best suited to satisfy the needs of every resident who will live in this development. The following pages will give the reader a general impression of the neighborhoods where each of the sites are located (Figure 3.1).

DESCRIPTION OF SITES

Site number one is a seventy-six acre parcel of land on the northeast periphery of Ann Arbor.

The parcel sits in the Northbury/Chapel Hill neighborhood, a well maintained blend of subdivisions, apartments, and condominiums. Plymouth Road, the southern boundary of this neighborhood, is lined with shopping centers, office buildings, and research facili-

[Haworth co-indexing entry note]: "Retirement Community Site Evaluation." Nicklowitz, Michael, and Kwang-Sun Choi. Co-published simultaneously in *Journal of Housing for the Elderly* (The Haworth Press, Inc.) Vol. 11, No. 1, 1994, pp. 37-50; and: *University-Linked Retirement Communities: Student Visions of Eldercare* (ed: Leon A. Pastalan, and Benyamin Schwarz) The Haworth Press, Inc., 1994, pp. 37-50. Multiple copies of this article/chapter may be purchased from The Haworth Document Delivery Center [1-800-3-HAWORTH; 9:00 a.m. - 5:00 p.m. (EST)].

FIGURE 3.1. Location Map–Ann Arbor

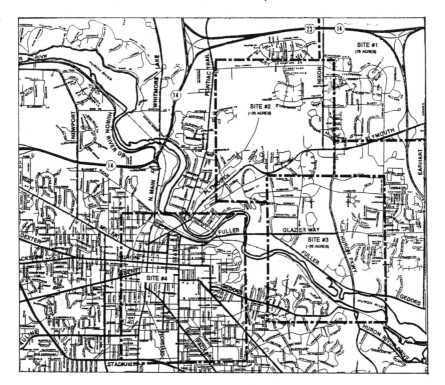

ties. Directly to the south of the parcel is Chapel Hill, a development of town houses, condominiums, and single family dwellings. About half of Chapel Hill consists of senior citizens. The remaining majority is made up of university students and staff. To the west, part of an undeveloped wetland is soon to be Oakwoods Park. Across Green Road and to the southwest lies Sugar Bush Park, a thirty acre green space with barrier-free walking trails.

- prices of homes in this area range from $110,000 to $210,000 and up.
- the median income per household is $40,000 to $60,000.
- the number of households with children ranges from 16% to 30%.
- the number of renters in this neighborhood ranges from 25% to 50%.

Site number two is a less than twenty-six acre site on the north side of Ann Arbor.

The parcel sits in the Traver/Willowtree neighborhood. This area is dominated by apartments, including Willowtree, Willowtree Tower, Parc Pointe, Parkway Meadows (which includes a group of senior citizen buildings), and Traver Ridge. The terrain in this neighborhood is extensively hilly with a network of ponds and streams that generally work their way into the underground storm sewer system. This parcel of land is bordered on the west by Leslie Park golf, a full eighteen hole public golf course covering 150 acres. To the north of this parcel and beyond a hardwood tree line lies Traver Ridge Apartments, a 210 unit complex built in 1972.

* prices of homes in this area range from $125,000 to $230,000 and up.
* the median income per household is $25,000 to $40,000.
* the number of households with children ranges from 16% to 30%.
* the number of renters in this neighborhood ranges from 75% and up.

Site number three, owned by the University of Michigan, is a large wooded parcel of land over 100 acres, of which twenty acres are being considered for this project. This site sits in the North Campus neighborhood, between the VA Hospital and Huron High School. To the north is Glazier Way and to the south is Fuller Road. The hilly glacial land is quite manicured but retains many wooded, undeveloped patches. Student housing in this area creates many densely settled neighborhoods. Directly to the north across Glazier Way lies Arborcrest Cemetery. To the west is a handful of older homes accessed off Oakway. These homes are owned by the University and have been earmarked for demolition to provide additional parking for the VA Hospital. To the northeast is a scattering of custom homes accessed off Glazier Way. These homes are well buffered from the road and each other. In the middle of the parcel of land is an overflow parking lot for the VA Hospital. To the south of the site lies Furstenburg Park, bordered by the Huron River. Furstenburg Park is a twenty + acre park designated as a nature area.

It is still not determined which part of this parcel will constitute the twenty acres, and because of other numerous proposed developments associated with this site, it is still uncertain if the University is willing to permit this parcel to be developed for this project. For the purpose of this study I will include the evaluation of this site for comparative reasons.

- prices of homes in this area range from $150,000 to $400,000 and up.
- the median income per household is $10,000 to $25,000.
- the number of households with children ranges from 31% to 45%.
- the number of renters in this neighborhood is greater than 75%.

Site number four is in the heart of the city near the newly expanded Ann Arbor Public Library on William and Fifth. This parcel of land is an existing parking lot in the Downtown neighborhood. "Most of the Downtown area lies on a plain between Defiance and Fort Wayne moraines. When the Huron-Erie lobe of the Wisconsinan glacier was in place 13,000 years ago, the Huron River was diverted to the west and flowed through the center of town toward Saline, leaving a flat lowland area in its path." Refer to the Topographic map of Ann Arbor. This area is now made up almost entirely of commercial developments. In the past decade this area has seen a regrowth of housing, some new developments such as Sloan Plaza and One North Main, and much rehabilitation of upper story apartments. Over half of the people living in this downtown area live by themselves and only 9% of the residents are over the age of sixty. This is an extremely active area with a plethora of shops and restaurants within a five minute walk.

- the median income per household is $10,000 to $25,000.
- the number of households with children is less than 15%.
- the number of renters in this neighborhood ranges from 50% to 75%.

EVALUATION OF SITES

In essence, a look at the surrounding environment at each of these sites is an important part of this study. "Where environmental choices are available, residents tend to choose those that match their ability level." For this reason I will now look at each site from a users point of view. Given the profile of the resident, active and retired at age 50 and up, I will assume that the sphere of activity may vary greatly from one resident to the next. If I own and drive a car I can set my sphere to easily involve all of Ann Arbor and many surrounding communities. Once I lose that ability to drive I must depend on other modes of transportation in order to maintain my sphere of activity.

Other modes of transportation may include taxi cabs, public buses/shuttles, trains, bicycles, walking and wheelchairs. Based on these ideas I will examine each of the sites by sweeping a quarter mile radius and then a half mile radius from the site and examine what amenities fall within this range. The half mile and quarter mile distance indicates a range considered to be a reasonable walking distance from the site for an active resident. The maps on the following pages describe some amenities offered within this range; 1990 aerial photos, and a topographic survey have also been included to better visualize the surrounding developments for each of the sites (Figures 3.2 through 3.9).

Site one, although secluded somewhat from the public sector, does offer Sugarbush Park. This park has areas for basketball, tennis, volleyball, soccer and bike paths. I'm not suggesting that a senior soccer league is a strong potential, but this park could provide one with an active area, as a sense of visual stimulus. The South Main-Huron Parkway Bus Route passes through the half mile radius, however, the pick-up area is nearly a half mile from the site and for the length of walk in front of Chapel Hill on Green Road, no sidewalk currently exists.

Site two maintains a moderate activity level with a variety of retail shops within or near a half mile radius of the site. A new walkway/bike path is under construction along the west side of Traverwood Drive; this would provide an easy and scenic access to Plymouth Road. Plymouth Bus Route along Plymouth Road provides stops well within the half mile radius. This site has the potential to provide a circuit of nature trails/walking paths within its boundaries and perhaps into Leslie Woods to the southwest.

Site three offers very little in the category of retail amenities, however, the Huron River Bus Route provides a stop within a quarter mile radius of the site. To the south of the site, within a half mile, a network of bike/walking paths parallel the Huron River through Furstenburg Park and Gallup Park. The University of Michigan North Campus is also accessed easily from this site.

Site four, being in the heart of the city, offers the greatest selection in the way of retail, cultural, transportation, and other miscellaneous services. On the other hand, the site offers many negative qualities such as limited area to develop, that is to say, any development on this site would have to be vertical. Crime is also more intense in the central business district as opposed to outside the downtown area. This is confirmed by the Ann Arbor Crime Report (July 1990-June 1991). Activity level in general may be a source of overstimulus, providing little if any areas of retreat.

Bicycle transportation is becoming a popular mode of transportation. City surveys have found that more than half the residents of Ann Arbor own a bicycle and half of these bike owners ride at least once a week. Among the 60 and over age group an impressive 20 percent classed themselves as bicycle riders. See 1991-1992 City Guide Ann Arbor Observer.

FIGURE 3.2. Area Map—Site One

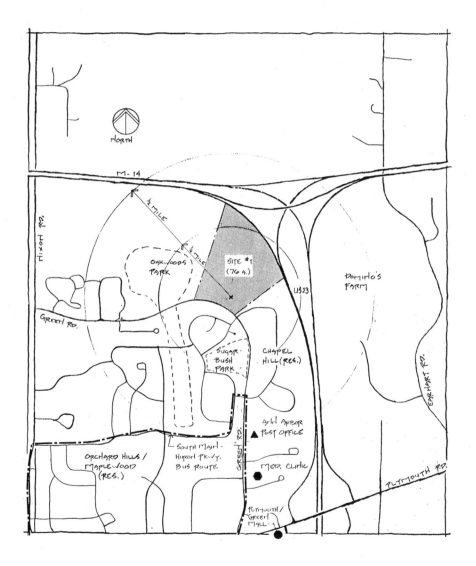

FIGURE 3.3. Aerial Photo–Site One

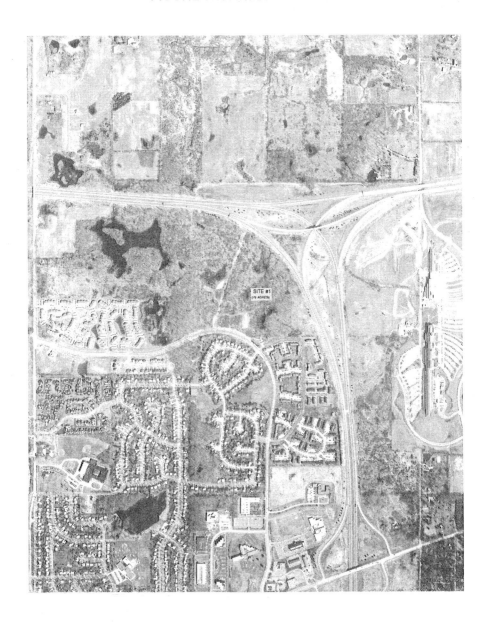

FIGURE 3.4. Area Map–Site Two

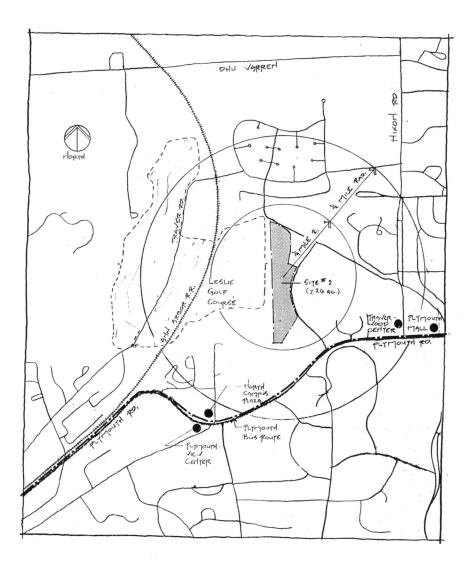

FIGURE 3.5. Aerial Photo–Site Two

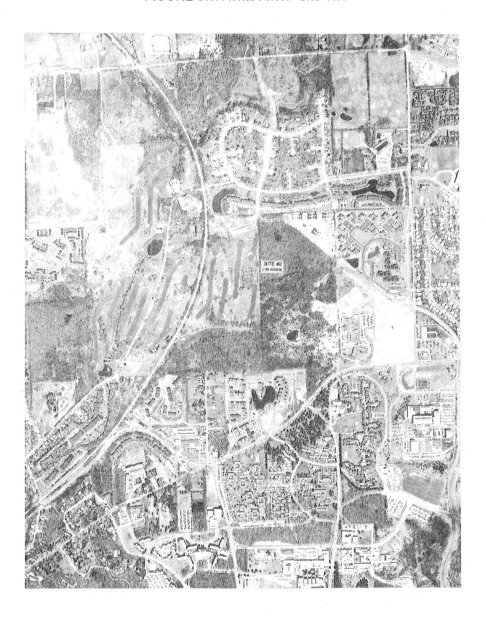

FIGURE 3.6. Area Map–Site Three

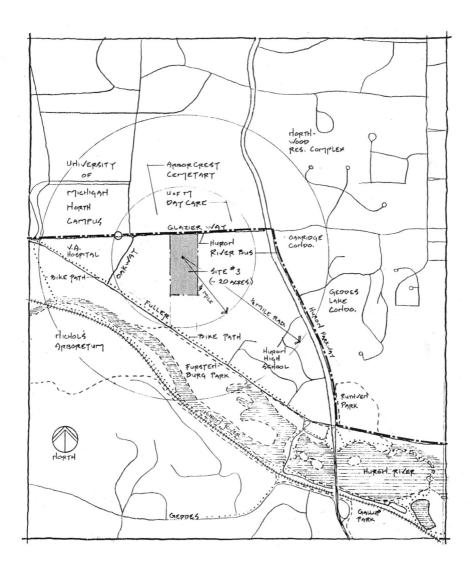

FIGURE 3.7. Aerial Photo–Site Three

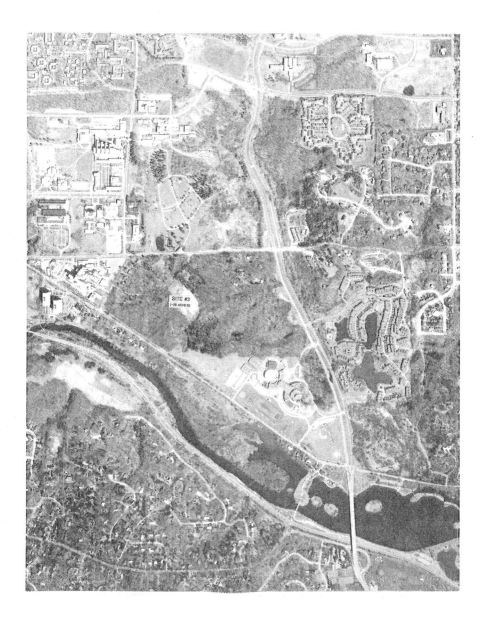

FIGURE 3.8. Area Map–Site Four

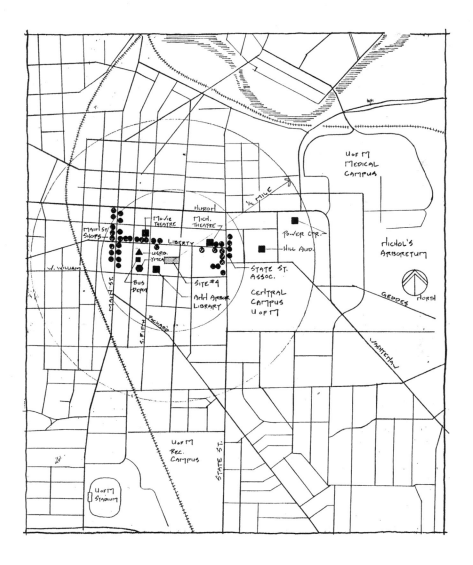

FIGURE 3.9. Aerial Photo–Site Four

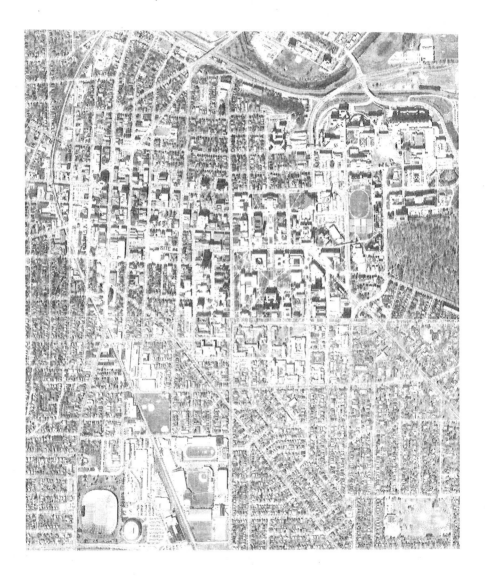

Public Spaces and Common Areas

Daniel Koester

THE ORIGINS OF RETIREMENT HOMES IN AMERICA

As an introduction to a discussion of public spaces within modern retirement communities, this paper will explore the historical development of retirement homes. The negative views often associated with retirement homes throughout this century has its roots in the period between the Civil War and World War I. The elements within American society which together created the legacy equating terms like "custodial care" with retirement homes will be discussed.

The period of time between the Civil War and World War I marks a significant transition in America in all aspects of culture and society. The elderly in the antebellum period, for example, were looked upon with respect because they exemplified the lifestyle consistent with living a long, happy life.[1] By World War I, however, the elderly were characterized as being much more of a burden than an asset, being viewed as dependent and requiring ever larger amounts of societal resources. A transition in the role of the elderly in American society occurred over this time due to many overlapping factors. The factors to be discussed here include demographic, economic, and socio-political changes within the context of the municipal/community response to these changes.

Between the Civil and First World War there was an increase in the number of elderly in society, especially poor elderly. Whereas in

[Haworth co-indexing entry note]: "Public Spaces and Common Areas." Koester, Daniel. Co-published simultaneously in *Journal of Housing for the Elderly* (The Haworth Press, Inc.) Vol. 11, No. 1, 1994, pp. 51-65; and: *University-Linked Retirement Communities: Student Visions of Eldercare* (ed: Leon A. Pastalan, and Benyamin Schwarz) The Haworth Press, Inc., 1994, pp. 51-65. Multiple copies of this article/chapter may be purchased from The Haworth Document Delivery Center [1-800-3-HA-WORTH; 9:00 a.m. - 5:00 p.m. (EST)].

the antebellum period, frail elderly were primarily the responsibility of the family, their increasing numbers and lack of resources exceeded most families' ability to deal with this burden. It was noted that "for the first time in American history, the aged as a group became the focus of national attention; some of the woes of being old were perceived as 'social problems' demanding comprehensive remedies."[2]

Many social factors contributed to old age pauperism during this period. Very few employers offered a retirement plan or any form of financial security to their older employees. Many elderly simply ran out of money. As a result, increasing numbers of elderly were ending up in almshouses, not as a result of poor living and work habits; they were simply poor, old and ailing. They entered the almshouse as a last resort in order to receive badly needed food, shelter, and medical attention.[3] It was during this period that the need for social programs such as mandatory retirement were being developed.

Ironically, the socially motivated programs such as mandatory retirement which were instituted as a means of providing security in old age, had the negative effect of reinforcing an emerging societal belief that there exists a "distinct barrier between old age and the rest of society."[4] The rapid growth in the rate of American industrialization at this time supported a commonly held belief that youthfulness was a distinct advantage for contributing to societies' continued progress.

The increasing number of dependent elderly inhabiting pauper asylums in the late nineteenth and early twentieth century was also part of a demographic shift in America. In New York City, for example, the City Almshouse was renamed the Home for the Aged and Infirm in 1903.[5] According to one author, "Private asylums had [also] been established across the country, attracting once middle-class elderly who became incapable of providing for themselves. The New York City Almshouse proposal was part of a larger movement affecting the care of the senescent. As a particular institution, its policies mirrored widespread beliefs about the needs and abilities of its aged inmates."[6] This example reflects both the demographic shift and the acquired status of "inmate" that was part of the almshouse vocabulary and thus continued as the institution transformed itself into a Home for the Aged.

The almshouse population, prior to the twentieth century, consisted primarily of those who were insane or mentally ill, those who were deaf, mute, blind, or otherwise physically handicapped, petty criminals, and a certain number of frail elderly. These institutional facilities tended to assimilate the elderly into their existing model of "care" without any plan to meet the special needs of this population. The most significant change was that, in addition to warehousing people, a greater emphasis was placed on in-house medical care. The medical thinking of this time period promoted the idea that deterioration with old age was inevitable and incurable, suggesting that the frail elderly need only a place to rest and receive medical maintenance prior to death. Thus, the new retirement homes of the early twentieth century remained very closely aligned in style and character with pauper asylums.

The main problem with this model of care was noted in that, "there was no clear line between elderly persons admitted because of sickness and debility, and those institutionalized simply for shelter."[7] The belief that all old people are doomed to degenerate, and the general lack of informed research concerning the actual needs of the elderly in society, predisposed the acceptance of the architectural typology of the pauper asylums in many subsequent institutional facilities for the aged, a predisposition present even today.

The programmatic typology for these facilities includes such elements as patient (as opposed to resident) rooms, bedrooms having multiple beds (thus multiple occupants and reduced privacy), shared bathrooms and showers, centralized nursing stations, public address systems throughout, hard floors, shining institutional appearance, large open lounges with vinyl and tubular steel furnishings, and large, undifferentiated dining spaces. These environments are more conducive to efficient staffing and custodial care than to actual resident needs. This typology for nursing home design, in reality, does not adequately meet the needs of staff or residents.

Fortunately, old age pauperism today is not the problem it was in the early twentieth century. Additionally, retirement communities and congregate living environments have improved significantly since this period. However, we can still trace modern beliefs and prejudices about such things as "custodial" nursing care as inhibiting factors in people's willingness to confront the full range of needs and thus desirable services within a retirement community. It precludes, in some cases, the ability to think innovatively about home health services and individual autonomy in dealing with both acute and chronic illness in congregate living environments. This does not need to be the case, in fact, it is the designer's responsibility to confront these issues head-on in concert with the developer and future residents of a new facility of this type.

It is against this backdrop that we consider modern retirement communities and the opportunity to create supportive living environments that emphasize the needs and abilities of their residents, not the preconceived ideas of "turn-of-the-century," institutional-minded designers, bureaucrats, and health care professionals.

MODERN RETIREMENT COMMUNITIES– COMMON SPACES

The discussion of common spaces in retirement communities will be prefaced with an excerpt describing the development of a true communal life-style in Merrill Court, a southern retirement center. The history of this facility's development of community activities is informative as it reflects how its residents established opportunities, where there previously were none, to participate both inside and outside its walls.

> There was nothin' before we got the coffee machine, I mean we didn't share nothin' before Mrs. Bitford's daughter brought over the machine and we sort of had our first occasion, you might say. There were about six people at the first gathering around the coffee machine in the recreation room. As people came downstairs from their apartments to fetch their mail, they looked into the recreation room, found a cluster of people sitting down drinking coffee, and some joined in. A few weeks later the recreation director "joined in" for morning coffee and, as she tells it, the community had its start at this point. Half a year later Merrill Court was a beehive of activity: meetings of a service club; bowling; morning workshop; Bible-study classes twice a week; other classes with frequently changing subjects; monthly birthday parties; holiday parties; and visits to four nearby nursing homes.[8]

It is interesting to note that the events described above centered around an activity people were naturally drawn to, a coffee clutch. Also, the activity was located in an open lounge area where residents could "look in" for activity while ostensibly doing something else, such as getting their mail. These factors made it safe for residents to participate without any commitment or formalized structure.

In considering the broad range of services that can be incorporated in a retirement community, it is necessary to define the wants and needs of the user population. A tremendous amount of information about community service needs has been provided within the Design Statement for the U of M Proposal. As noted in the introduction of this statement, the intent of the project is to provide housing that "would provide a collegial setting with facilities and activities that could lead to a fuller life than would be possible otherwise. This will provide the opportunity for the residents to be involved in some intellectual or artistic activity."[9] The next section discusses the public areas which have been explicitly identified within the Design Statement.

UM PROPOSAL–PUBLIC AREAS

The Design Statement provided a basis for this research effort and included a rather detailed description of the types and characteristics of the common spaces desired for the facility. Some of the items received greater endorsement than others in this list, however, for the purposes of this research they will be treated with equal importance. Table 1 provides an outline of the common areas planned for the facility.

Prior to analyzing the specific spaces defined in the table, it will be instructive to consider the kinds and amount of public spaces within different retirement community types. Attempts have been made to categorize the various types of retirement facilities and their common areas and services as a means of creating a typology. The types range from Retirement Towns to more traditional nursing home facilities. The three types to be discussed here are those most closely aligned with the U of M Proposal and include: (1) Retire-

---

TABLE 1. UM Proposal–Public Areas

1. Central dining facilities
2. Areas of relaxation, recreation, education
   Large lounges
   Small lobby lounges
   Library
   Music area
   A shop
   Craft room
3. Health-related space for medical support
4. Circulation areas
   Lobby
   Delivery & emergency entrance
   Garden room entrance
   Hallways, Stairways, Elevator
5. Outside areas
   Flower and rock gardens
   Horseshoes, Tennis, Badminton
   Croquet, Volleyball, Shuffleboard
6. Other
   Mail room
   Guest rooms
   Extra Storage for residents
   Beauty parlor/barber shop

---

ment Villages, (2) Retirement Residencies, and (3) Continuing Care Retirement Centers or CCRC's.

According to Pastalan, "Retirement villages are intended to house a retirement and pre-retirement population in a secure setting offering a wide assortment of leisure and recreational activities. Retirement villages are not planned to be self-contained communities. Recreational and communal facilities and programs are prevalent. Indoor facilities typically include a clubhouse with rooms for meetings, performances, crafts, games, and an assortment of classes. Outdoor facilities include swimming pools, golf course(s), shuffleboard courts, and tennis courts."[10] The average size of the villages is ten times that of the U of M Proposal, however, the service structures are similar in that they cater to the more youthful and active population.

The second type to be discussed is the Retirement Residency;

again, according to Pastalan, these "small communities of older people [are] often housed in a single high-rise building. Besides apartments, retirement residences contain communal rooms and dining facilities where residents may be required to eat one meal per day. [They also] generally lack outdoor recreational facilities such as golf courses, tennis courts, and swimming pools. At the same time, their social programs and the indoor facilities . . . might include lounges, craft areas and/or game rooms, and multipurpose rooms. Planned programs, organized by resident staff, typically include classes, parties, lectures and excursions to places in the surrounding area."[11] This option tends to be marketed to the lower end of the middle class income range.

For elderly individuals who can afford and desire a more supportive housing option for retirement, one that includes a health care component, the third type or CCRC is a viable option. According to Pynoos, "Community spaces in CCRC's often include large communal dining facilities, libraries, crafts rooms and auditoriums. Many communities also have beauty and barber shops, post offices and banks, and convenience stores."[12] Like retirement residencies, according to Pastalan, "they rarely have facilities for active outdoor sports."[13] It is this type of facility that seems to be outside the needs and desires of the U of M Proposal due to the cost as well as consideration for the potential downsides of providing for a less able population of residents (i.e., those who require periodic health care services). It will be vital to consider fully the health care needs within the U of M proposed facility, the available community programs to support that need, and that portion which can be handled within the facility. Given the extensive health care services available in the Ann Arbor area, it seems prudent to take full advantage of available resources instead of recreating them in-house. To the extent that there may be some useful design ideas within the CCRC model, it will be discussed further.

The CCRC is probably the most recognizable descendant of the almshouse model of nursing home care. They usually have medical or hospital-like areas for individuals with more extensive health care needs. The division of common spaces usually includes rehabilitation facilities, as well as in-house medical and therapy staff. To the extent that CCRC's resemble the "archetypical" nursing home, it has been noted that, "residents normally have access to 12 distinct spaces within a facility."[14] These "archetypical" spaces are described in Table 2.

A number of parallels can be drawn between the common spaces indicated in Tables 1 and 2. In comparing Table 2 to Table 1, it may be advantageous, in the U of M Proposal, to think of the "therapy" areas as part of a larger health and fitness center instead of more "archetypical" therapy designations. Certain machines considered valuable for therapy may be purchased for this facility along with accommodating the fitness equipment placed in this area by the residents themselves. Recent studies have revealed strong associations with even low intensity exercise and improved health and well-being. This will be discussed in greater detail later in this paper.

With respect to common spaces in CCRC's, the most unsuccessful aspect is the single function use of many common areas. It is noted by Pynoos that in most design specifications, either by designers or others involved in the planning, these spaces tend to be unifunctional. The author contends, however, that "the facts are that spaces are multifunctional, serving many requirements–both designated and undesignated, and they will be altered by time and by changes in population."[15] As the designers of facilities of this type, there is a strong incentive to create flexibility in the environ-

---

TABLE 2. Common Spaces Within CCRC's

1. Patient-resident room
2. Lounge
3. Corridors
4. Dining rooms
5. Entrance areas and lobbies
6. Activity areas
7. Bathrooms
8. Occupational therapy areas
9. Physiotherapy areas
10. Beauty parlors and barber shops
11. Chapels and worship areas
12. Outside areas and the community

ment to facilitate change, customization, and multiple use by residents.

LOUNGES IN RETIREMENT COMMUNITIES

With respect to the U of M project proposal, the designation and use of lounge space is discussed in terms of large lounges for activities and small lounges, such as at the main lobby area, for more intimate conversation and relaxation. It is worth giving particular attention to the allotment and "designed use" of lounges within a retirement facility. In his Ph.D. thesis research of the post-construction evaluation of a retirement facility, Eric Osterberg observed the uses of lounge spaces by the residents.

> It was also found that sometimes residents preferred not to use spaces for their designed purpose. An example is that the residents all have comfortable TV "lounges" in their rooms. Anyone who wants a TV nowadays can have one. The function that TV lounges in nursing homes served in the past, when televisions were expensive and not many residents owned them, are perhaps no longer appropriate. In another lounge area in this same facility, one that was located along a corridor, it was found that these lounges were frequently filled with wheelchair and walker storage.[16]

These examples indicate that the designed use of a space is not always successful for its intended purpose. Additionally, the practical needs of the resident population can evolve and change with time. From a functional and cost perspective, the facility designers must consider carefully the division of personal versus public spaces. When public space is not utilized for its intended purpose, such as the TV lounges mentioned previously, the space may be better off being added incrementally to the private spaces of the residents. Pynoos asks the question, "Why can't the square footage requirements devoted to lounge space on a per capita or bed number basis be translated into socialization areas in corridors or in the patient rooms themselves where they would be of potentially more benefit?"[17] In the article, *Building in Residency Throughout the Facility Plan*, the design and use of lounge spaces is further discussed.

> In the current state of the art of building nursing homes, lounges must be regarded as the single greatest failure as a concept. Typical lounges usually result in one or more very large areas devoted to socialization, relaxation, and contemplation, but not really accommodating any of these activities. The large open space that usually characterizes the lounge is counter-productive to intimate communications between two people or small groups. Many activities will be taking place at the same time, and because of rigid scheduling. Lounges can either be isolated or enclosed, with access through a doorway or passageway, or they can be open areas near an entrance, at the intersection of hallways, or in a space not unlike a harbor just off a corridor to one side or both sides. The isolated lounge is less attractive than the open lounge because there is less potential for activity that can be passively observed. The open lounge provides access to high activity levels for passive observation, but it does not permit effective interchange among the occupants of the space. Lounges need to be smaller and more accessible to the whole population within the nursing home. This means transferring space devoted to lounges to patient residents rooms. In truth, it means abandoning the well-worn concept of an isolated multifunctional room, which does nothing well and is a great waste of money.[18]

This rather negative view of lounge space raises more subtle questions about open and closed spaces and the opportunities and problems associated with each. In the example presented earlier at Merrill Court, the open space where the coffee pot was located created a tremendous opportunity to the residents that otherwise may not have been realized. Initially, in the U of M Proposal, *the need for the passive observation of activity will not be as great as the planned attendance at events and activities.* Still, as a means of meeting new people and combating loneliness, the ability to have space for passive enjoyment of others is desirable.

DINING ROOMS

Another major area that is well developed within the U of M Proposal is the dining facility. A number of details of the dining facility have been considered that will positively affect the space. These suggestions include the idea that the dining spaces be modulated with movable screens and planter boxes in order to provide greater privacy and intimacy in these areas. This point was addressed by one author with respect to noise that can be a problem in large, unmodulated dining facilities. "Dining rooms can be very noisy [making] conversation indistinguishable from background noise for many of the elderly. Dining rooms seem to be designed from the standpoint of seating as many people as possible without fully considering the effect of passage, serving of food, and the ability to penetrate beneath table surfaces and egress backward from this position."[19]

Other details which must be resolved early on in the design process are the furnishings that will be used in the dining area. It has been suggested that dining chairs for the elderly to be selected should have arms on them to ease getting in and out of them. With this in mind, when chairs do have arms, it is important that they be able to penetrate beneath the apron of the table so as to be out of the way for both residents and staff to perambulate within this area.

Table design is another factor which must be resolved and requires decisions about planned flexibility of the dining area to seat large groups or a more static arrangement. It has been noted about dining tables that, "a four-position table provides a configuration that places everyone in view of one another [and] a round table allows approach by a staff member from any side for serving a no discriminatory seating positions."[20] Round tables cannot be put together as readily as square or rectangular ones for larger groups. On a day-to-day basis, the number of people at a table should be between two and six people in order to ensure that the dining experience remains intimate; using small tables is more conducive to conversation.

HEALTH CARE AND FITNESS FACILITIES

Although it is not a major part of the U of M Proposal, health care facilities must be considered and levels of in-house and community services that will be available. Much of the literature reports the extent of services available in retirement facilities, particularly those related to health and recreational services.

For any retirement community, there is a need to create a hierarchy of wants and needs for public spaces. The various service attributes of a community can be considered in terms of their type and quantity. The various service combinations and arrangements are discussed in the following excerpt.

> Health, recreation/leisure, social, and commercial services and facilities. Outdoor recreation facilities consists primarily of golf courses, swimming pools, tennis courts, and marinas, whereas indoor facilities range from meeting rooms to club houses and libraries. Services can also be represented by programs such as arts and crafts, classes, and outings to local area attractions. A commercial service can vary from a shopping center with an array of stores to a gift shop or a privately operated snack bar in a single building. Health care and outdoor recreation are viewed as the most important dimensions of the service attribute, and together with a combination of other services (social programs and facilities, commercial, housekeeping, maintenance), form five basic service packages found in retirement communities:
>
> 1. extensive health, outdoor recreational, and other services;
> 2. limited health and extensive outdoor recreational and other services;
> 3. limited health, outdoor recreational, and other services;
> 4. limited health, outdoor recreational services with an extensive array of other services;
> 5. limited outdoor recreational services with extensive health and other services.[21]

One aspect of the planned retirement community is the desire to include people who are primarily active, self-sufficient, contributing members of the community. A question for the designers of the facility is, can spaces be created that encourage healthful living? To what extent does the "management" want to create opportunities for the residents to participate in fitness and health related activities and education? Some justification for making this an important part of the design program is provided in the next section.

Many retirement community builders will market various health care services so as to attract both elderly retirees and the young elderly who are sensitive to the fact that their needs will change over time. The number of continuing care retirement centers should expand to meet the demands of the longer living elderly who will seek a protective environment guaranteeing them continuing health care. The issue is addressed in the U of M Proposal, "we hope to develop a 'health room' where supplies and equipment for limited physical examinations can be provided for use by visiting nurses, physicians, or therapists."[22]

The following statements, taken from a recent article in *The Gerontologist*,[23] discuss the needs and benefits of exercise specifically for women, however, the information is also applicable to men.

- Evidence is rapidly accumulating that physical mobility is a critical survival need for the elderly and it seems clear that older women have much to gain from improving their exercise habits.
- Possibly the most important outcome of physical activity is stress reduction, because it is linked to other benefits such as better sleep, muscle relaxation, positive mood states, and improved self image and self concept.
- An important support to psychological health is clearly the opportunity created by exercise to socialize, to play and have fun with peers, form new relationships, and develop a community spirit with other elderly people.
- There is no medicine that can help overcome the range of conditions for which exercise has been prescribed: obesity, depression, diabetes, arthritis, hypertension, coronary heart disease, menstrual cramps, migraines, smoking, and other states.
- It does seem clear that a commitment made to an active lifestyle, even if it doesn't extend life, does play an important role

in maintaining one's mobility and physical independence–keys to maintaining quality of life.

- Hand in hand with the search for better life-styles to accompany aging is the concept of a life-span approach to education, which suggests a need for continuous adult education, particularly with respect to health promoting behaviors.

CONCLUSION

This paper has reviewed several aspects of common spaces within retirement communities which can serve to inform and inspire architects and designers. The information should be valuable to the research team with respect to the design of common areas, as they proceed to the next phase of design development for the proposed retirement community.

REFERENCES AND BIBLIOGRAPHY

1. Achenbaum, W.A. (1978): *Old Age in a New Land*. Johns Hopkins University Press, Baltimore, MD.

2. Ibid., p. 90.

3. Haber, C. (1951): *Beyond Sixty Five*. Press Syndicate, Cambridge, England.

4. Achenbaum, p. 108.

5. Haber, p. 82.

6. ibid, p. 82.

7. ibid., p. 87.

8. Hoschild (1961): Communal Living in Retirement Facilities. In *Old Age in America*, Lang, G.E. (Ed), H.W. Wilson Co., New York, NY.

9. Design Statement (1991): University Senior Faculty, p. 1.

10. Pastalan, L.A. (1985): Retirement Communities. Generations, IX(3), Spring, p. 27.

11. ibid., p. 28.

12. Pynoos, J. (1985): *Options for Middle-Upper-Income Elders*. Generations, IX(3), Spring, p. 31.

13. Pastalan, p. 29.

14. Pynoos, p. 42.

15. ibid., p. 42.

16. Osterberg (1977): Ph.D. Dissertation, University of Michigan, p. 56.

17. Pynoos, p. 54.

18. Koncelik, J.A. (1976): Building in Residency Throughout the Facility Plan. In *Designing the Open Nursing Home*, Dowden Hutchinson & Ross, Inc., Stroudsburg, PA, p. 53.

19. Pynoos, p. 54.

20. ibid., p. 55.

21. Marans, R.W. et al. (1984): Retirement Communities. In *Elderly People and the Environment,* Altman, I., Lawton, M.P., Wohlwill, I.F. (Eds), Plenum Press, New York, NY, p. 65.

22. Design Statement, p. 3.

23. Obrien et al. (1991): Unfit Survivors: Exercise as a Resource for Aging Women. *The Gerontologist,* Vol. 31, No. 3, pp. 347-357.

Housing for a Retirement Community

Madelyn Wilder

INTRODUCTION

A recent study by the American Association of Retired Persons shows that 86 percent of senior citizens want to remain in their homes until they die. As the population ages, demand will soar for architects who specialize in renovating homes to suit an elderly person's special needs and in designing long-term-care facilities to be as homey as possible. A health designer might remodel a bathroom so that a wheelchair could roll into the shower, for example, and replace doorknobs with lever handles, pull curtains with electronic drapes and lamps with a central lighting system. The floor plan of a nursing home might be drawn to group bedrooms around a communal sitting room.

Residential quality is of great, if not primary, importance. The key to designing toward openness in a health care facility for the aged is to focus upon the needs, general requirements, and desires of this population from the beginning of the design process. One important facet is to express appropriate concern for the residential qualities of the physical environment, as well as the health care and service aspects of the setting. It would be better to overstress residency vis-à-vis health care in the general qualitative atmosphere in order to prevent institutionalization from becoming predominant esthetically and attitudinally (Koncelik, 1976).

[Haworth co-indexing entry note]: "Housing for a Retirement Community." Wilder, Madelyn. Co-published simultaneously in *Journal of Housing for the Elderly* (The Haworth Press, Inc.) Vol. 11, No. 1, 1994, pp. 67-76; and: *University-Linked Retirement Communities: Student Visions of Eldercare* (ed: Leon A. Pastalan, and Benyamin Schwarz) The Haworth Press, Inc., 1994, pp. 67-76. Multiple copies of this article/chapter may be purchased from The Haworth Document Delivery Center [1-800-3-HAWORTH; 9:00 a.m. - 5:00 p.m. (EST)].

CHARACTERISTICS OF THE ELDERLY

Older Americans are a complex group of individuals who are impossible to strictly categorize. Each person ages at a different rate with varying consequences and levels of adjustments. Research, however, has been able to identify common experiences which people encounter as they grow older. Although one cannot monitor these changes with a definitive schedule, general trends are evident to which the designed environment should respond.

The successful development of a residential community for senior citizens is contingent upon accurately defining and understanding today's elderly population. Elderly housing is more than just physical shelter, the societal implications must be realized and addressed. The comprehensive housing development should be responsive to its surrounding neighborhood, but also to the facts and realities of the aging process. It is not possible to change society's preconceived ideas on the elderly overnight. However, it is a reasonable objective to create an environment which enhances the resident's life satisfaction. Providing opportunities for the elderly to establish a viable role for themselves is essential.

To meet this goal, encouraging community support will aid in eliminating the social isolation and alienation of the seniors. The housing solution should respond to both the physical and social needs of the older populace. Special care must be taken to plan for varying degrees of resident dependency. Each elderly person will have different requirements for care; some desiring complete independence while others will want continuous skilled care. Flexibility in the facility will allow the housing complex and available services to adapt to the individual needs of the residents.

In addition to the obvious medical services, the physical environment will have a great impact on the aging person. The designer should incorporate the potential for future increased support in each individual unit without compromising the independent and ambulant senior. The designer can target three levels of support. The resident with complete dependency will require skilled medical care and continuous observation. Others will need some medical services but will be able to handle most of the daily activities alone. These residents, possibly handicapped or with limited mobility, may desire minimal support services such as housekeeping aid, common dining facilities and out-patient medical care. The independent senior will require limited out-patient health services and can benefit greatly from a social network and the assurance of good medical services when needed.

INTERIORS FOR THE ELDERLY

Here is a quick look at some interior design implications for the elderly.

- The environment is becoming active in services for aging people. The environment and its objects do more than 'look good'; they must work well and communicate feeling (i.e., comfort, welcome, high quality). Looking 'good' may mean feeling familiar or may involve inviting a frail person's confident use.
- Texture is used in more ways. The idea of the 'touchable environment' is interpreted literally as one that communicated warmth and coziness.
- Environments are more varied. Rather than picking one style, motif or color pattern for a whole building as one would in a hotel, individualization and personalization are being taken more seriously.
- Environmental design is becoming part of the organization's image. The facility that emphasizes fitness and wellness has chairs selected for action and motion. The facility with a keen activity center incorporates lighting to accommodate close work.
- The process of design is changing. More people are participating, more information is available, more products are being developed. It's truly worth asking for what you want: furniture manufacturers, lighting engineers and designers are competing to respond to industry requests.
- Good design is 'seamless'. It does not look 'odd' nor draw attention to the infirmities of people. It attracts young and old equally well. And good design works as a system rather than as a single object, color or room (Hiatt, 1986).

CREATING AN ENVIRONMENT

One of the most remarkable differences between a long-term care facility and a short-stay, acute care setting, should be the use of objects. In acute care, the focus is appropriately on the admitting condition. In long-term care, we are concerned with the whole person: physically, psychologically, socially, and spiritually.

A home-like environment is one where personal objects are within reach and view, where they stimulate thinking, provide comfort, and offer hints as to one's interests and identity. While there may be a few people who have never had many possessions, who live more in their imaginations, far too many institutions presume that they can accept a person without taking in some of his or her trappings. Part of the difficulty has been that objects must be stored and cleaned. Few bedrooms adequately provide vertical spaces: shelves, picture moulding, or ceiling hooks which would allow items to be kept without getting in the way.

By encouraging room personalization, a retirement facility can do much to convey its personality to the public. The variety in possessions may be more effective than any particular wallpaper or institutionally-devised color scheme to convey a unique and 'caring' message. Elevator lobbies, corridors, and even living rooms of some apartment residences and health care facilities have been effectively decorated with furnishings from the residents (Hiatt, 1984).

Beyond the more direct design implications of the built environment, additional design principles which address the needs of the aging should be incorporated to facilitate a successful living arrangement. These components include:

- Design elements which lessen the feeling of being institutionalized and increase the ease of negotiating the environment.
- Providing the potential for exploration through the use of various forms, textures, colors, and activities. The aim is to keep residents active and motivated.
- Permit residents to choose own role and level of participation in community affairs. This freedom supports the independence of each person and increases general life satisfaction.
- Providing the individuals with the sense of 'Home-Like'.

Achieving these design goals requires good insight and knowledge of the elderly population on the part of the designer. Additionally, the concern and involvement of the community is crucial. There is potential for the local community to take advantage of what the elderly have to offer, i.e., a day-care center for children. It seems to me that today's youth could benefit from what the elderly community has to offer. There are some general characteristics of older Americans which should be considered when planning a senior housing complex. Some of the basic needs of the elderly person include:

- Participation in community activities of own choice and at own pace.
- Availability of good public transportation to counteract the decreased level of mobility of the elderly.
- A neighborhood atmosphere without physical or social isolation.
- Encouragement of autonomy and independence of the resident through the provision of convenient necessary services.
- Reasonable distances and topography to allow resident to negotiate the environment safely.
- A secure environment to ease resident's physical and psychological anxiety.
- Design should convey feeling of permanence rather than transitional shelter since 90 percent of those over 65 years do not change residences.

The careful development of appropriate design guidelines results from the thoughtful response to elderly residents and their diverse needs. As people reach various levels in the aging process, increased degrees of support are required to allow the aging person to perform the basic daily functions. The needs are as different as the people who live in any one community. Flexibility is the key in providing adequate care for the elderly while recognizing that the type and amount of support will change continuously. The ultimate goal of elderly housing is to provide the necessary physical and social support to further the independence and enhance life satisfaction of the residents.

HOUSING ENVIRONMENTS

Elderly housing should strive to create an environment which will contribute to the maximum physical and mental functioning of older persons. Goals are followed by their rationale and possible methods of achievement.

Encourage Independence. The ability to care for one's self promotes a sense of pride and increases self-esteem. The design of elderly housing should allow persons to live as independently as possible in spite of the reduced sensory and mobility levels that accompany the aging process.

- Provide barrier-free design to accommodate persons using wheelchairs and walking aids.
- Install safety features such as handrails and non-slip surfaces in an unobtrusive fashion.
- Provide repetitive visual cues through the use of graphics, color or planting to aid in orientation.

Encourage Social Interaction. An older person's social contacts are reduced due to retirement from work, death or poor health of friends and less involvement in their children's lives. Opportunities to establish new social contacts should be provided.

- Provide spaces for informal social contact. The prime locations are entrance lobbies, mailboxes, and alcoves interspersed along corridors.
- The potential for social interaction will be increased if the size of the development is not greater than 300-400 units. If living units are arranged in smaller clusters the opportunities for informal social contacts will be even greater.
- Group activity spaces should be located adjacent to one another in an 'activity hub'. Visual access between them will provide opportunities for informal interaction.
- Activity rooms should be small in scale with furniture arranged to encourage small group formation.
- Outdoor spaces may also be designed with seating and informal gathering spaces to encourage interaction among residents.
- Participation can be stimulated by providing a variety of activities in a visible location.

Encourage Interaction with the Community. The residents should be provided with the opportunity to continue their previous roles in the community to prevent feelings of isolation and social disengagement.

- Provide residents with access to shops and services either by proximity or a transportation service.
- The on-site amenities may serve the neighborhood elderly as well as the current residents.
- The use of community services and amenities is preferable to the 'island' approach of providing everything on-site.

Minimize Institutional Characteristics. Buildings with an institutional appearance or feeling will segregate the elderly from the community and encourage dependent behavior.

- Building mass should be minimized by creating smaller clusters of units. Familiar housing materials such as brick, wood, fabric and carpet should be used.
- Minimize rules and regulations. Allow residents to participate in decision-making.
- Avoid mandatory meal services. Each unit should have a kitchen so residents have the option for personal or group dining.
- On-site medical care facilities are convenient but should be minimal and unobtrusive.
- The size and scale of the development should fit harmoniously into the neighborhood.

Allow Opportunities for Individual Choice. Aging is a process which slowly closes out options to the individual which in turn creates stress. By providing options, the individual can better maintain their physical and mental health and a general sense of well-being.

- Provide a variety of types of living units such as one or two bedroom independent apartments as well as congregate arrangements.
- Avoid mandatory services but provide a variety of accessible services.

- Permit residents to furnish their dwelling units to suit their personal tastes.
- Residents should have control of the heating and cooling system for each individual unit as well as operable windows.

Provide a Secure Environment. The elderly are concerned with their personal security. This will affect the degree of their involvement and social interaction. Unfortunately, the fear of attack and robbery causes many elderly persons to isolate themselves.

- Install emergency call systems in individual units and at various public areas in and around the buildings.
- Ensure safe pedestrian access to neighborhood services.
- Avoid mixed low income and elderly housing which tends to have a higher crime rate.

HOUSING TYPES

Independent Retirement Housing Units are self-contained apartments designed for active or young elderly people. In urban and metropolitan areas they are usually mid-rise buildings: approximately eight stories. Typically, their minimum size would be one hundred residential units. The more economic size would be about two hundred units, and the maximum three hundred. The economy of scale comes through the distribution of management services, purchasing and so forth. In rural communities a similar type of housing has been sponsored, largely through the Farmers' Home Administration, and is usually single-family dispersed cottage-type housing. The scale of the units, because the communities are smaller, ranges from twenty-five to one hundred units.

Congregate Housing developments provide some communal services in addition to the basic independent housing units. This housing includes communal areas, help with cleaning, shopping, and has communal dining facilities. It includes most types of assistance with independent living, short of direct personal care. Congregate housing demands a high level of servicing and staffing, so management costs are higher.

Personal Care Housing/Assisted Care recognizes that there is a need for personal care housing where frail or older elderly people can receive personal care and assistance with dressing, washing, etc.

Skilled Nursing Home is the building type that cares for the elderly person in need of both personal and medical care and support. Skilled nursing care involves supervision by a physician and intermediate nursing care involves supervision by a licensed nurse. Their size normally ranges from 120 beds, which is usually considered to be the minimum economic operating level, and increases in 60 unit increments (based upon the number of beds per nursing station), with 240 bed units probably being the most economical to operate. The scale of the facility is very much tied to management practices which attempt to realize economies of scale through a consolidation of experience.

Life Care Communities are the most recent and certainly the most sophisticated development in housing for the elderly and first started in the early 1960s. The normal population runs from 300 to 400 residential units. The facilities provided are usually divided into four types of units.

1. Independent living: these tend to be bungalows or apartments for the active elderly.
2. Self contained apartments: these are combined with communal facilities to provide meals plus some social activities.
3. Personal care accommodation: this usually takes the form of single bedrooms and is intended for frailer, older elderly.
4. Nursing home facilities: the accommodation here would be similar to that of personal care, with the exception that medical supervision and care would also be available.

A common feature of life care communities is also to include a continuing care contract which covers the remainder of a resident's life. The ratio of self-contained apartments to nursing care units varies from one apartment per nursing care bed to just over four apartments per nursing care bed. This very much depends upon the management policy and market need of a particular location. Typically, the nursing care unit would have 60 beds (Valins, 1988).

HOUSING CATEGORIES

There are a wide variety of housing types serving elderly persons today. The great majority of the elderly do want to maintain their independence and, as a result, live in single family homes. As individuals become less mobile, however, the level of personal choice may be directly dependent on the proximity of support systems and the degree to which services can be delivered into the home. Failure to develop these services adequately can only lead to premature institutionalization.

It is true that many older persons do thrive in age-congregate living facilities. Unfortunately, there is very little semi-independent housing available to satisfy the needs of middle and low income people. They are forced to live in retirement hotels, with their children, or in nursing homes.

BIBLIOGRAPHY

Gelwicks, Louis E. and Newcomer, Robert J. *Planning Housing Environments for the Elderly.* Washington, D.C.: The National Council on Aging, 1974.

Hiatt, Lorraine G. *Conveying the Substance of Images Interior Design in Long-Term Care.* Contemporary Administrator, April 1984.

Hiatt, Lorraine G. *Effective Trends in Interior Design Planning Facility Design.* Provider, April 1986.

Koncelik, Joseph A. *Designing the Open Nursing Home (Part III).* Stroudsburg, 1976.

Lucas County Senior Complex: Retirement Housing Research Group. APRL–University of Michigan.

Rowles, Graham D. *A Place to Call Home.* Handbook of Clinical Gerontology. New York, 1987.

Valins, Martin. *Housing for Elderly People,* Great Britain, 1988.

Community Sense

Melissa K. Lucksinger

Melissa. I wanted to start by telling you some of my basic concepts and ideas, and how I formulated them. These ideas have become the basis of my project, the core of what's happening. It all started a year ago when we started this class on retirement communities. Benny and Lee started slowly chipping away at all my ideas of old people. After a year of this class I've definitely rethought things and come up with my own ideas on the issue of aging and how people live while aging. So first of all I'm going to go through some of these concepts.

From the beginning I focused on the community and the elderly. This has become my focus because my feeling is that through a communal existence, through living in a communal environment, everyone, but especially people that are aging, will have a more positive life, will be able to do more because of the support that they

[Haworth co-indexing entry note]: "Community Sense." Lucksinger, Melissa K. Co-published simultaneously in *Journal of Housing for the Elderly* (The Haworth Press, Inc.) Vol. 11, No. 1, 1994, pp. 77-97; and: *University-Linked Retirement Communities: Student Visions of Eldercare* (ed: Leon A. Pastalan, and Benyamin Schwarz) The Haworth Press, Inc., 1994, pp. 77-97. Multiple copies of this article/chapter may be purchased from The Haworth Document Delivery Center [1-800-3-HAWORTH; 9:00 a.m. - 5:00 p.m. (EST)].

get in that community. These ideas started in the paper I wrote for this class, and from this paper they've evolved into something you see here.

To start off, I have some quotations and little pictures to help explain my ideas. These two drawings are the basis of my ideas (Figures 6.1 and 6.2). The first one is about the university setting. The university setting becomes, if not a fountain of youth, then surely a context for continued growth. The university is a place where most of us have first lived in any form of community with relatively homogeneous people. Elderly people who are associated with the university can continue their spiritual and intellectual growth. It's not just a dead end. It's no longer retirement at 65 and "go out to pasture and leave us alone." "We don't want to see you anymore." This is about bringing the elderly back into society and letting them continue to contribute. Elderly have a lot to give. My other main concept is the idea of aging in place and what aging in place really means. One of the ways of aging in place as it exists today is a continuing care retirement community. You have different buildings that have different levels of care and each time you require another level of care you must physically pick up and move to a new place. But this is considered as aging in place because you're kind of in the same radius. Well, I don't particularly buy that. I think that there is a better way we can do that. I think that by equipping each individual unit with the facilities so it could be converted into an assisted living apartment you can take care of the individual in a different way.

This diagram shows the main support system and the minor support systems. I realize the logistics of this is definitely difficult but my idea on aging in place is to decentralize the services and the support. In this way you get the caregivers closer to the people so they don't have to drive long distances for the care. You don't have to drive all the way back out here to give someone care. I've developed these larger communities, and each community has a node, these squares being the nodes. That is where I propose that the main support services for each community will be located (Figure 6.2). And then there will be some form of mobile care that can go out from each one of those nodes to service the people in this general community area.

FIGURE 6.1. Designing Elders' Utopia

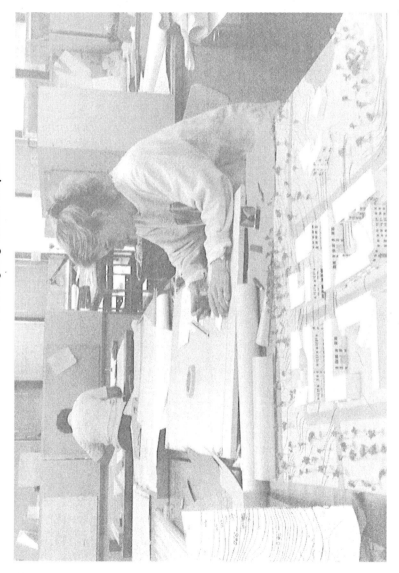

FIGURE 6.2 Site Plan

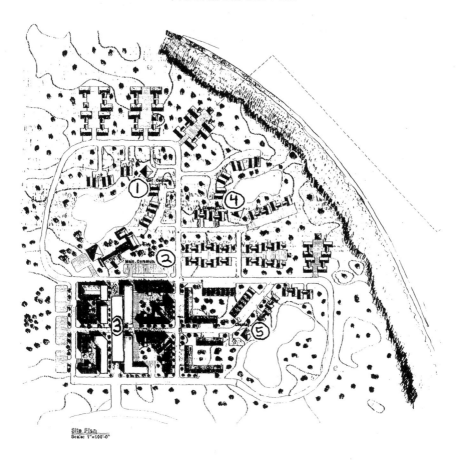

Site Plan Legend

1. Cluster Center
2. Main Community Center
3. Main Street

4. Cluster Center
5. Cluster Center

It comes back to the question why community living and why should I move out of my single family home that I own–and I've lived here for 30 years–into this retirement community. My idea is that by living in a community you get over the sense of isolation that so many elderly feel they have. A lot of people live alone and their ties to the community used to be work. When they retire they become separated from the rest of the community. So my idea is that living in this more homogeneous community with other retired people who have a lot in common can bind the people together. And by binding with each other they can rely on one another for support. In the design of the community I think it's important to encourage this interaction. I realize that I can't design something and say okay this is going to happen here, but my idea is to provide the opportunity for interaction by clustering units of housing, and hopefully people will interact in daily life. Each little neighborhood would have its own little grocery store. So people get up in the morning, get their paper, get their orange juice and they can see people coming and going.

The bottom cluster is showing a very important idea for me. This is the idea of choice. From what I've seen in a lot of nursing homes is the lack of choice. "It's time to get up and take a walk around the room." "Okay, well, now it's 10:30, it's time to do this." People are told what to do. And if they don't want to go to sleep it doesn't matter, it's time to go to sleep. So, my idea here is about choice. There's a variety of activities and there's also a link to the rest of the community, to the campus, to Ann Arbor, to downtown, the library, linking all these things together. So people have the choice how much to participate in the community life. So, there's a choice of participation there and you can be involved with as much or as little as you like. Once again, the idea of community is that by living together with other people around one can get support and therefore it enables people to live on their own. And then there is the unique relationship in a university setting, that is the intergenerational activity that one can have. Here I have a little diagram that has the children and it says, "I want to be a financial wizard, an artist, a teacher, a doctor, a lawyer" and over here you have the elderly and they have already experienced these things. They've achieved this. They have a valuable experience to share with other people. Through a university setting people can share ideas and they can start to break down stereotypes each group may have of the other.

To move on to the next board, my focus here has been on the development of what I call Main Street (Figure 6.3). This is the

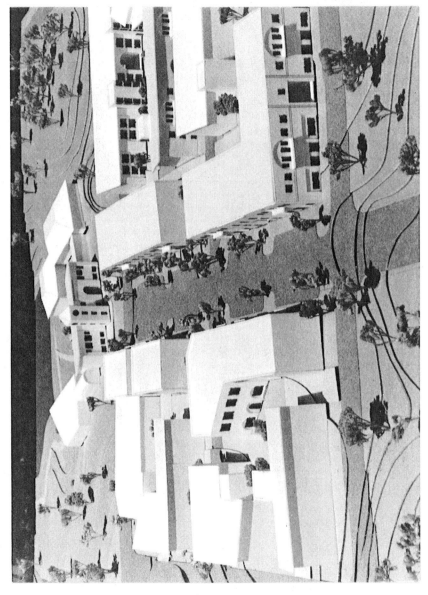

FIGURE 6.3. A Model of Main Street

entrance to the community. When you enter right here you have immediately this kind of a dense urban area. You're entering straight down this street and the idea here is to provide services to the people because where this community is located is near Plymouth Road, but not close enough for walking distance for anyone of the residents there. The idea here was to bring some services into the neighborhood and get people from the area to come and use the services as well. So there's shopping, there are some doctors' offices, and other commercial services right here on the bottom floor of what I call Main Street. And then up above on the third floor you have apartments. I realize that this is rather a dense area but my idea was kind of a European community where you have lots of interaction with people. Everything's very close within walking distances. You don't have to get in your car to drive, but then again you can if you choose to.

At the end of the access of the main street is the community center which is the heart of the community itself. It has services like auditoriums, lecture halls to relate to the University, a library which is on-line with the university library system. You can go down to the library, but you can access things from the community also. Here you have activity areas and rooms and also a restaurant.

Each dwelling unit is equipped with a kitchen, but there are a variety of dining options. This one right here would be the major dining area for the community, more of a commercial dining area. This block right here is represented in the model (Figure 6.4). You can enter through various points here into this more privatized courtyard area. A visitor would probably come in through this main entrance here. This is the lobby entrance and then this area back here is a dining area with lounges on either side. The idea in the design of this is that you have basically more of a glass wall on the inside to view the courtyard, to bring the outside in. In some of the nursing homes I've seen, I have noticed big problems with light. Lack of light seems to make things look very institutional. So I wanted to try to bring the outdoors inside. Each individual unit here has its own balcony. So there is that outside, you can go outside if you'd like to. And the balconies are arranged in a way where two units more or less share a balcony. There's a division between them but the idea, again, is to promote interaction. Personally I live in an

FIGURE 6.4. A Floor Plan of a Typical Housing Cluster

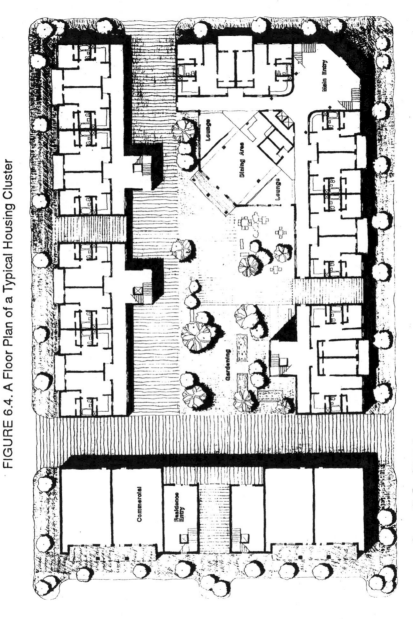

apartment complex and the only way I've met my neighbors is on the balcony outside, cooking out. People don't seem to meet their neighbors these days. It's just something that I wanted to change.

Entering into these units there is a variety of entry nodes. The idea of this is so that you don't have to go through the main lobby if you don't want to. You don't have to walk in the same way everyone else walks in. You can choose your own way and that way you begin to identify with the people that share the node. This node has two apartments on each floor, is three floors tall, and it has its own entry. So, hopefully these people will meet in the elevator and in the seating areas out around here. This courtyard, I see as being a fairly vibrant place. It's got areas for gardening, seating, some green space. I see it as a place where people will want to go and sit and take things in and watch the activity. Then there are also places throughout the site where more dense urban activities can take place. I'm also proposing to have a walking trail going around the edge of the site. I figured I can take advantage of the scale of the site and create as much activity and outdoor use as possible (Figure 6.5).

This is a section through the main community space. These different levels where you can look down and see what's going on enable you to see people all the time. It helps to create this feeling of interaction and community. This section is through a typical bay of the housing unit. It shows the roof slanting in to start to bring the scale more down to the human scale. This is one thing I've dealt with a lot on this project. I wanted everything to relate to the human scale instead of overpowering it. In the elevations right here, for example, is this arch form. The arch represents the idea of living. You can see the arch in the residential areas. I see it also as more of a human scale factor.

N. Levine. How do you handle the automobile associated with this? Is this pedestrian only?

Melissa. No, it's also for automobiles. That's something that I fought with desperately because my initial ideas were to have this pedestrian because cars make our spaces ugly. But, once I started to think about this, I thought that the car also gives a lot of mobility and autonomy. So, I developed underground parking within these dense urban areas and these streets were designed for people and for

FIGURE 6.5. Sections Through a Typical Housing Cluster

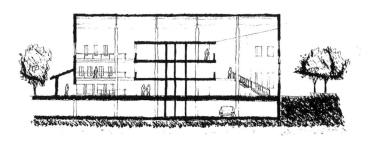

Entry/Lounge Section
Scale: 1/16" = 1'-0"

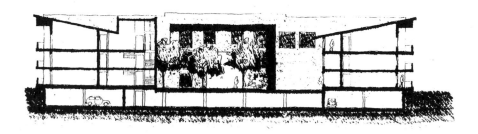

Living/Courtyard Section
Scale: 1/16" = 1'-0"

cars. There are trees planted around the edges so hopefully they will create a buffer zone between the cars and the people.

You can choose where to live. You can live downtown in this urban area, and you can come out here to more of the apartment-like styles, or out here to more spacious living quarters. These represent the cobble paved court in between the houses, so the cars and the people walk and drive on here. This is an example of turning the typical American front yard and back yard inside out. Where the back yard is usually the place for activity, now I'm making the back yard more of a paved environment for interaction and then they have all this surrounding green space.

D. Cinelli. I have two questions. How many total units do you have on the site?

Melissa. I have 375.

D. Cinelli. Total acreage covered?

Melissa. It's about 76 acres.

D. Cinelli. The second question I have is based on Lee's comment at the beginning. He made a comment about the missed opportunity with most CCRC's in this country being aligned with a university. How do you feel your CCRC has addressed that, not only as adjacency of the same town, but your major concept about how this is different than any CCRC in the country?

Melissa. My idea of it being more of a little city in this dense urban area and the fact that there are choices offered. Not everything is ramped. There are some places where it would be steep or harder to walk. You can take that route or you can go the other way. In relation to the University, I've obviously gone over and over in my mind about what it is that makes the University unique. And I think of walking across campus at Michigan and the Diag and all the people out there is just kind of the aura of learning. What I've determined is the relationship of the people in the buildings and nature and the way they are interacting.

H. Naimark. Would you conceive this as a rental community or purchased condo kind of thing?

Melissa. My idealistic idea, would be to own it. Because I think if you own something, it becomes your home. I think that renting my apartment doesn't make it home. I think ownership is the ideal. But once again, I'm not real sure about the logistics of that.

H. Naimark. The second question is what level of independence will the residents be when they first enter this community?

Melissa. I would see them as very active and vibrant. They can come in and be the go-go crowd and then as they age they can still remain in their house. And they can have facilities to support them so hopefully they can still maintain a certain amount of activity.

G. Tipton. Can you talk through how exactly you envision that happening? I mean, you struck on a main theme that people do like to hold onto home, and not be forced to move to another environment because their physical condition has changed. Central to that if they maintain the home that they moved into, is bringing services to them.

Melissa. Right.

G. Tipton. Can you talk us through that–they're starting out as very go-goes and eventually they'll slide, perhaps, to a no-go situation. How do you envision these services being delivered?

Melissa. I envision that the initial design of the apartments to be what I've seen called a universal design where things are movable. Where there are places for grab bars and hand rails that can be attached but they don't necessarily have to be there. Because I think that immediately stereotypes it as an old person's place. But I see all facilities being able to adopt to physical changes. There would have to be a core provided in the initial design so that these services will be able to be plugged in. For instance I can see a nurse that might come in and help the person with the activities of daily living, etc.

G. Tipton. The more intense needs such as the full nursing care would also be delivered to the individual unit?

Melissa. Yes. But, I think that full nursing care would be up to a point. I don't think that complete nursing care for bed-ridden patients would take place here. I'm not sure that I agree with the idea of a nursing home. Because if you're sick enough, then maybe you belong in a hospital and not in a nursing home.

N. Levine. Recognizing logistics of your site, taking into consideration that you're contiguous with single family residential on either side and your peripheral edge where the curve is taking place is your noise problem. Ecologically you've looked at the site's constraints relative to change of topography, and you picked up on some of the potential areas such as the lake areas, and really set forth a central node with secondary passive nodes, with your little villages (Figure 6.6).

Melissa. Right.

N. Levine. There are 375 units within the context of your program. Your central node area being the commercial or more active public oriented area would feed your community but also you have to realize that what is contiguous and related to that has to support its activities economically as well. Did you take that into account that your neighborhood is really enlarged by what you have contig-

FIGURE 6.6. Aerial View of Main Street

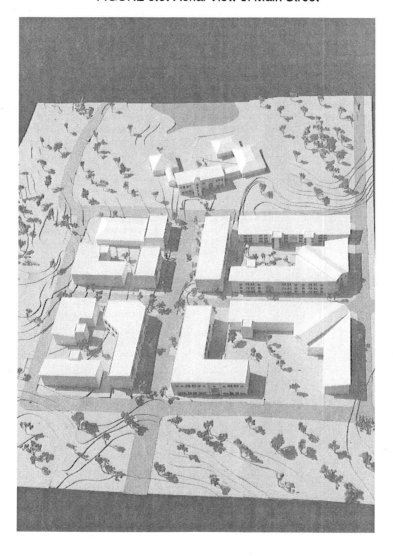

uously? And also what would you call intergenerational interface on the site as what you are dealing with in family structures?

Melissa. Actually I see the larger community being a great benefit because I think that's where you get more interaction from a younger generation or from different people. It's not always the same faces. By having single family housing around here, you can have children here and you can have younger couples. In these areas you have a fitness center, a store, a library, a park. These things can be your intergenerational draws. In the community center I envision also day-care being offered. I tried to create this public interface. I think that the surrounding community helps support this, because on its own I don't think that the commercial spaces would support itself. The larger community is needed to support it and hopefully that interaction will make a richer community.

N. Levine. Do you think that the vehicular circulatory system should have only one means of entrance or egress or should they be interfaced with the single family areas that are contiguous? Would this help you?

Melissa. Just having one entrance I see as being a benefit in terms of safety, to feel safer. And by having one secured entrance you help monitor who's coming and going. So I think that that's helpful. While I want public interaction I'm not so sure that this guy out here wants Mr. Jones from two miles away to come and play in his back yard. So I think that there is a reason for having just one main entrance.

G. Tipton. I'd like to make a couple of observations. One to talk about is the whole notion of the University relationship. We've worked on a project which literally adjoins a university. It was not sponsored by the university, but it immediately adjoins it. All the concepts of having this interrelationship are there. But it hasn't happened. None of that has happened. All the things that you would hope could happen, haven't. But yet the immediate adjacency is there to make it happen. Yet we worked on another project where they foster a relationship with a much more remote university where all the services of that university are broadened, educational programs are broadened to that retirement community and actually some of the staffing is brought from some of the younger people coming to the university. And many of the residents go to the university for classes as well. So the whole notion of making a success almost has more to do with the philosophical relationship between the institutions than even the physical relationships. That's one aspect. The other thing, you seem to have done a really excellent job of including the concept of choice as being part of what makes one's life experience a positive one in a home-like setting. You have a choice to go to a corner drugstore, grocery store. You can go to one place or another. It's not locked into one kind of living which is reminiscent of one's home. I want to bring that back to aging in place though, because it's one of the things that we've experienced in our practice in the reality of doing these communities. As much as we would like to foster the notion of having the person who moves into this community as their home, they age in place. Other people that surround them have chosen also this retirement community to live. They see their neighbor aging in place and their physical condition changes whereas their perception is that they haven't changed that way. In the ideal world you would hope that there would be continued support from one neighbor to another. Unfortunately very often what we've seen, it doesn't. There is a pressure from the better conditioned elderly on the administration of the community to provide an alternative setting for the less able person. In this design where persons are aging in place in that unit that they've selected there may be another problem. Because there are common facilities there, but those facilities are less easily accessible for those people as they age. They have to go outside to get to them. They may become, inadvertently, isolated in their unit and become even more shut out from the community than you originally hoped they would be. Because they are not getting the support from the neighbors. I'm talking real broadly.

Melissa. Right. It can backfire. I understand what you're saying.

G. Tipton. I mean, it's just something that I think as we approach designs, we like to foster this whole notion. But it's a real issue of aging in place. The sociological relationship of the person's image of themselves when they see their neighbor's condition deteriorating. I don't want to sound like such a pragmatist, and such a realist, but I've seen that in my own practice. I think it's a commendable goal but I would just worry that as individuals age in place they may become very isolated in that kind of unit.

D. Cinelli. I think that people because of market requirements are trying to package a segment of the adult population. I think they've done a real disservice to the aging community by not letting someone be able to bring a wheelchair or a walker to a part of a retirement community. Marketing people say: "Well, it's the resident council who really says they don't really want to be reminded about their own mortality." I think in a way the direction has been preordained. If you look at a lot of European models there's a lot more intergenerational type environments that they buy into culturally. I think as Americans we've sliced everybody in society so thin.

Melissa. That's exactly what we've studied about the Scandinavian experience. I was trying to relate those ideas more to an American context. After looking at the Scandinavian facilities I came up with this pedestrian approach. I felt that this is the way to go. I can get rid of the cars. But in America the cars are necessary.

J. Hoadley. I think that one of the things that we have to be realistic about is what triggers an individual to begin to live in a retirement community. My experience has been that typically a health episode of some sort has begun to reduce the individual's choices. People are very much attuned to a reduction of choices and if we pick an individual up and flop them into an environment that is totally different from where they came from, it becomes a vast mental torture for them. I think we need to take a look at where these people came from when we design these facilities. I think that in order to trigger the vibrant senior to moving in, you're probably talking about somebody that hasn't had that episode yet. In this case we need probably to have more active type things in the project in order to really successfully draw the person who just wants to live there because it's a great environment.

G. Tipton. One thing about those who do elect to move to a retirement community. Typically they have been those that plan ahead, that anticipate the event that hasn't yet happened. And that's probably an excellent relationship with the university because those folks tend to be better educated and have thought through the process of what aging will have in store for them. A retirement community provides the opportunity to have that all the way thought through and have the various levels of care provided for them. The question is in what place is that care provided and do you have to move people from one place to another. Can you successfully provide the care in the chosen place? Because they don't want to pick up and move.

D. Cinelli. I just wanted to make a comment about what Lee said in the beginning. It seems to me that the missed opportunity really is that this project should really be a part of housing in the university. I mean, I would have loved to see what the University of Michigan diag looks like. There are certain things that sort of subliminally hit us as we use a university over a number of years, of what makes it a special place. The arcades, the distances, the courtyards, the Law School Quad, all of those kinds of things are special features which make that up. I think that what you have done on your site plan is really talk about these elements. But I think you have a really missed opportunity. I mean I like the fact that when you drive in there's this vista down the main street, the community center is at the focus point, that there is urban living, suburban living and rural living, because that's where your constituents are coming from. But I would have liked to see more elements from the university. I would have liked to be able to have this co-mingling. The Pines Retirement facility is sponsored by Davidson College in Davidson, North Carolina. What they've done is they've made all of the programs accessible to the elderly. They can audit classes for free, but there's no particular reason why the students and the faculty would ever want to go over to the Pines. I think that introducing town retail is a great idea. I think the ability that, I don't have to eat in this dining room but there's a little cafe that I can go over here and sit and have a cup of coffee and exchange views, is the kind of idea that Lee was talking about. The ability as a retired faculty member to talk with students. This is the real program element that you're missing. I don't think you've pushed it far enough.

Melissa. No, I haven't. I agree with you and my main focus for the project was on this area. I wanted to plan a site with these ideas I had about the aging in place and the services. I wanted to see what I could come up with but my focus has been on this area. I agree.

G. Tipton. One of the things that makes a university life so vibrant is the diversity and the range of choices that you have. And to that extent I think this project strives to achieve that. In that sense this project is conceptually similar. It doesn't have the overall functionality that directly mimics, say, the University of Virginia which in some ways has an interesting parallel to a retirement community with their connecting walkway to a central community building. But when done in a direct mimic (and it has been done, not by us) it has left the participant without that sense of success that you have in the university setting. Perhaps because the range of diversity and choice you have in university setting isn't there in the retirement community.

Melissa. I struggled also with the scale. When I first got this site plan, I was a little overwhelmed. I didn't really realize how big 76 acres was. So I took maps of the University. I found out that you can place about every single major space in the University on this site.

G. Tipton. One of the things I think you've done nicely was to relate the community center as a center for this whole site. Whereas it is one axis with the main street of your urban center, it is skewed to set up a relationship to the suburban and rural settings of the site, which is good. It says: "This is the center of this entire community, not just of the urban part." I think that to push it to the overlap with the University perhaps functionally or in some other way means also to push it into the direction of how one would age in place and still have the range of choice and diversity. This can be the next step I would want to take this to.

N. Levine. In defense of what you have done planning-wise is that you're working in a context of a specific site. What you've done at the site, you've looked at what you can do with the person that is aging in place. And speaking environmentally we're looking at the passive environment, the active environment, those environments that are in between and what we're dealing with as far as human beings as they age through the continuum of life. The idea of choice throughout the context of the site itself is the most important element; you're dealing with behavior. Because as we age we have many factors to deal with and the location of each entity within the context of that site. You're asking yourself a question: "What will this individual do as he ages, or how do the constraints of aging impact upon that person as he ages within the context of the site itself?" The logistics of the site says: "Well, somewhere down through the aging continuum, I want to make that distance a little bit shorter for that person to walk to that community center. I want to enable that person to make the choice to either walk through the so-called main street or the possibility of picking up the little van that might take them to the University." The options are there. You had a site located with many constraints. You had to answer the questions such as the noise problem. You've built a major buffer along the highway. You've actually oriented your buildings perpendicular to that noise factor to say that I've recognized it. As we age we know that many things are going to happen to us. They happen differently with every human being. And as you look at the site itself, how did you really get into that and really address that? The site itself is important as to how we utilize it. As our world begins to shrink we want to be able to have those activity nodes become more and more available to us because we don't want to fall into the trap to be lost within the context of one's home and be forgotten.

T. Hille. My question has to do with the types of buildings that you've introduced here. You have the apartments, you have the rural housing. Most of these people will be coming here from which of those?

Melissa. I would think most of them would be coming from single family homes.

T. Hille. That's what I'm curious about. I would expect that.

Melissa. My idea on that was why would you move from your single family home to another single family home?

T. Hille. Well, I'm not sure. Perhaps because it's smaller or because it's part of the scheme of things.

Melissa. Right.

T. Hille. I would think that the idea of going to an apartment, let's say, may have functional justifications. It may have social justifications as well. It might be easier to make contacts. But looking at the types themselves, I would expect that there would be some people who would prefer a single family house and in fact a duplex is a funny compromise in a way. You could probably easily rearrange those as detached houses and really all you'd lose is nothing. And psychologically I think it is a big difference.

Melissa. I definitely see your argument. My idea was to create the proximity thinking that if people are closer together, hopefully they will interact. But, like you said, there is a point at which you don't want to hit them over the head. I'm going to have to agree with you. I think, maybe, the next step would be to provide another level of choice. So, if you want to live in a single family house you can.

T. Hille. But just to carry that up to the scale of the site, I would also be wondering about the way you'd then organize those elements. To me the first thing that would come to mind would be straight kind of blocks instead of blocks of houses the way the town is designed. That's what Ann Arbor is all about. It seems to me that the model that you're looking at more closely, with the exception of the little central town area, is really more like a condominium development than a neighborhood development of traditional sense of town.

Melissa. When I started off on planning the site, I went immediately and laid my grid down. I thought that this is going to organize me, it's going to get me going. And then I picked my grid up and I still had a grid on the site. So as I started developing it I tried to push away from the typical block to give it a little bit more freedom to move around. So that's how the development went.

T. Hille. I think the organization of those various sized components of the house, of the block in the neighborhood can take a number of configurations. You could look at it again, as a village which is much more responsive in America. I'm less concerned about if we can get to the perimeter, I think the big issues do come up. I appreciate that you minimize the exposure to busy traffic ways that create noise and that sort of thing. But the single access, to me, is the hallmark of that development and I think that you're really caught here in a paradox of wanting to connect to the town and yet somehow being afraid that the issue of security is keeping you really interactive and yet the idea to me is very attractive. Especially in a university town which is a relatively safe place to live that could you have more of this which would mean that you would have to connect to the surrounding area more directly. But ultimately you isolate yourself and you're right back to the same problem that you create a ghetto. So you use your commercial center. You try to draw people in but instead you isolate them because of the physical form condition that you set up by isolating yourself on either side.

Melissa. You think that more entry to this central core area would have helped?

T. Hille. For instance if you should locate the commercial area as a carrot to get people to come into the community. I would think that putting it on the commercial strip and then beginning to use that as my buffer that would protect the neighborhood which sits behind it, that's a standard pattern for towns everywhere. Commercial street that are an edge condition that inside of that protected homes with less traffic, for example. But that is one approach. But as soon as you start to isolate that element in the side, you at least pull it over to an edge, that helps. You don't have to put it dead center, you'd be in worse shape. These are just sort of planning issues that I don't consider in any priority. They really have a lot to do with your design.

Melissa. Thank you very much.

Residential Quality

Madelyn Wilder

Madelyn. I'll start with my concept as it is broken down here into the constraints, ideas, and solutions. The obvious constraint was the noise factor of the highway and how do the people relate to it. As you can see there are some hills that we had to contend with (Figure 7.1).

We didn't want to have the housing look like warehouses. People don't want to live in a nursing home type of situation. I asked myself why do people want to come here? The individuals who live out in the country in physical isolation, why would they want to live in a community-type situation? This is a picture of the neighborhood on this side and there's another little apartment structure on this side. You will get an idea of the buffer situation.

In the beginning of this semester I started the project at the same time with Melissa. She was concentrating on the community part of the development and I put the emphasis on the housing.

I chose for my commercial development a pedestrian street keeping the cars to either side of it. The main entrance coming in and then breaking up into the housing section of the division. The services would be maybe small cafes, shops, and smaller grocery stores. I also envisioned places where people can do research or teach classes or lecture halls, or similar amenities. We were trying to figure out how we could get the students to come in. One of the ideas was to create a facility for people when they flood the town

[Haworth co-indexing entry note]: "Residential Quality." Wilder, Madelyn. Co-published simultaneously in *Journal of Housing for the Elderly* (The Haworth Press, Inc.) Vol. 11, No. 1, 1994, pp. 99-119; and: *University-Linked Retirement Communities: Student Visions of Eldercare* (ed: Leon A. Pastalan, and Benyamin Schwarz) The Haworth Press, Inc., 1994, pp. 99-119. Multiple copies of this article/chapter may be purchased from The Haworth Document Delivery Center [1-800-3-HAWORTH; 9:00 a.m. - 5:00 p.m. (EST)].

FIGURE 7.1. Concepts Board: Constraints, Ideas, Solution

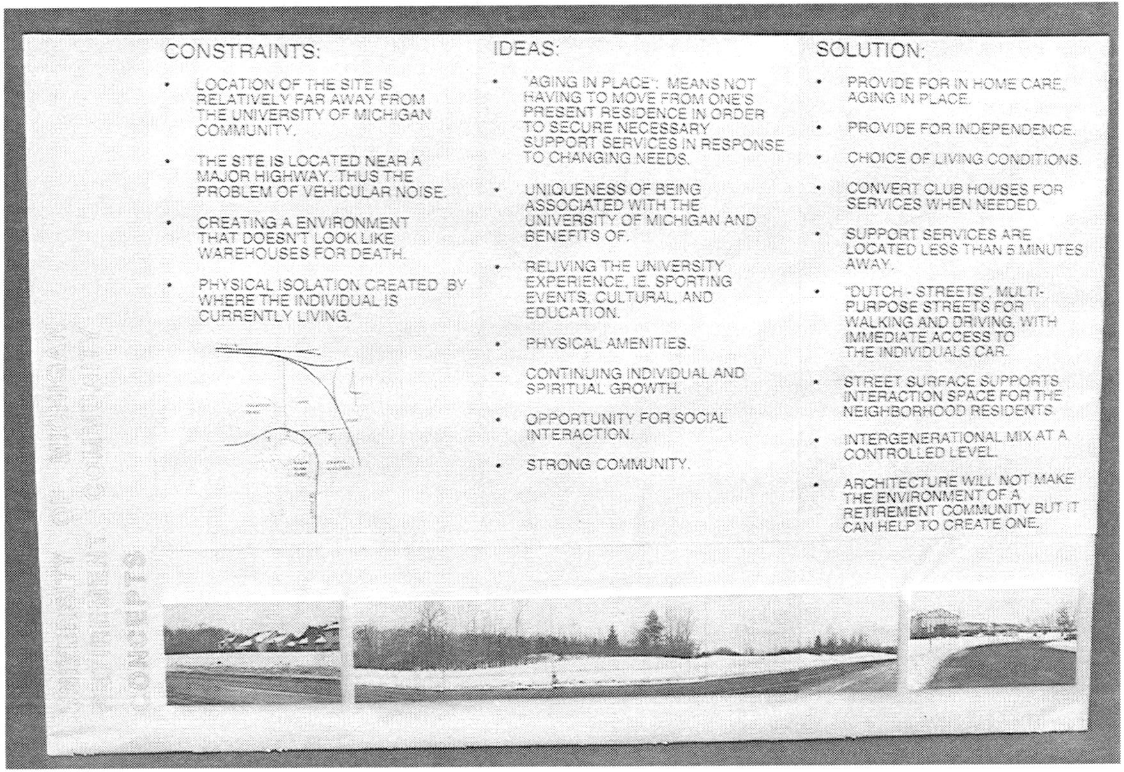

CONSTRAINTS:

- LOCATION OF THE SITE IS RELATIVELY FAR AWAY FROM THE UNIVERSITY OF MICHIGAN COMMUNITY.

- THE SITE IS LOCATED NEAR A MAJOR HIGHWAY, THUS THE PROBLEM OF VEHICULAR NOISE.

- CREATING A ENVIRONMENT THAT DOESN'T LOOK LIKE WAREHOUSES FOR DEATH.

- PHYSICAL ISOLATION CREATED BY WHERE THE INDIVIDUAL IS CURRENTLY LIVING.

IDEAS:

- "AGING IN PLACE" MEANS NOT HAVING TO MOVE FROM ONE'S PRESENT RESIDENCE IN ORDER TO SECURE NECESSARY SUPPORT SERVICES IN RESPONSE TO CHANGING NEEDS.

- UNIQUENESS OF BEING ASSOCIATED WITH THE UNIVERSITY OF MICHIGAN AND BENEFITS OF.

- RELIVING THE UNIVERSITY EXPERIENCE, I.E. SPORTING EVENTS, CULTURAL, AND EDUCATION.

- PHYSICAL AMENITIES.

- CONTINUING INDIVIDUAL AND SPIRITUAL GROWTH.

- OPPORTUNITY FOR SOCIAL INTERACTION.

- STRONG COMMUNITY.

SOLUTION:

- PROVIDE FOR IN HOME CARE, AGING IN PLACE.

- PROVIDE FOR INDEPENDENCE.

- CHOICE OF LIVING CONDITIONS.

- CONVERT CLUB HOUSES FOR SERVICES WHEN NEEDED.

- SUPPORT SERVICES ARE LOCATED LESS THAN 5 MINUTES AWAY.

- "DUTCH - STREETS", MULTI-PURPOSE STREETS FOR WALKING AND DRIVING WITH IMMEDIATE ACCESS TO THE INDIVIDUALS CAR.

- STREET SURFACE SUPPORTS INTERACTION SPACE FOR THE NEIGHBORHOOD RESIDENTS.

- INTERGENERATIONAL MIX AT A CONTROLLED LEVEL.

- ARCHITECTURE WILL NOT MAKE THE ENVIRONMENT OF A RETIREMENT COMMUNITY BUT IT CAN HELP TO CREATE ONE.

100

for a football game or other sporting event that could stay within this community. This place can serve alumni or relatives coming to visit. Another idea was an adult day care center where the people could volunteer their time to take care of the neighboring kids in the area and the interaction resulting from that type of situation. Once we'll get into the housing I'll explain another intergenerational idea. Still I couldn't ignore the basis that I do need a strong community (Figure 7.2).

Once you get past this point, you get really into two types of neighborhoods with community centers being on the four corners of the area. I envision really this one as being a major type of center. My project is also using the aging in place type of idea. But I foresee here what happens to a person that needs a place to stay under supervision because of a broken hip, etc., a person that needs 24 hour care. I don't envision that in the houses themselves. I foresee part of this facility for somebody who could go there, recuperate, and then go back to their house rather than going out into a nursing home situation. This could be just a small clubhouse type atmosphere, a gym, a workout place. Maybe a place to go and play cards, or a meeting, a dance, social events, that type of thing. And also there could be a service outlet out of the same location. My idea is that a caregiver could get from here to the person in need within five minutes. To these neighborhoods you will enter from the insides of the courtyards. I envision most of the people in this area not having cars. These are small two-story apartment-condo type buildings. This area right here is enlarged in the model (Figure 7.3).

This was the focus of my project. I dealt with the Dutch street-type atmosphere where the street becomes a brick paving where you can walk on and you can drive on. All the major interaction of the people are in this type of area. But you also have the choice of a private area being in the back yard. The floor plans consist of two bedroom facilities with a living room and a kitchen and a one-car garage which could be converted. If you didn't have a car maybe you wanted extra space for a hobby workshop or that type of situation. Within these small subdivisions there are smaller clubhouses. When people move in, maybe they're younger, in their fifties or sixties and they don't need the services. Maybe at that time this is just the clubhouse. As the people age in place this can be converted

FIGURE 7.2. Site Plan

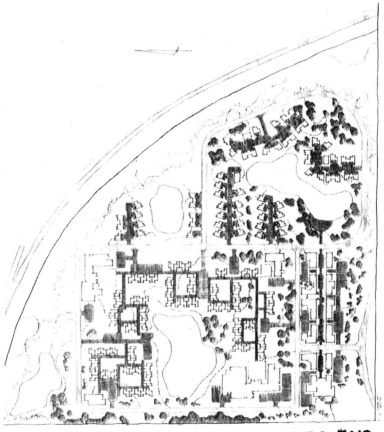

SITE PLAN
RETIREMENT COMMUNITY
UNIVERSITY OF

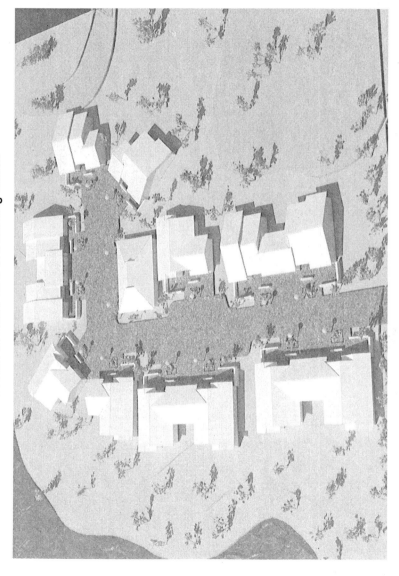

FIGURE 7.3. Aerial View of a Housing Cluster

to a small care center where a nurse can stay within the community and provide care to the people who need it. I was thinking that this could be a nice area for children. A place where a retired adult can meet with children.

L. Knight. So the main focus of the building would be to provide some kind of health care services?

Madelyn. I foresee a portion of it being a community center. Maybe there is a swimming pool or another activity. But yet the other half would be the health services.

L. Knight. There would be beds? Some people could stay there as long as they needed for recuperation?

Madelyn. Yes.

L. Knight. I think that, you might just add that. Because the reason why most people go into a retirement community is to have that insurance or maybe access to health care if they need it. They hope they won't need it, but the reason that a retirement community is so beneficial is that people have the access to service. People who enter retirement communities are planners in terms of their future. It's kind of like buying insurance, self insurance knowing that if you need the service it will be there. So I think it's great that you incorporated in your design that recuperative 24-hour nursing care for someone who needs it.

Madelyn. I don't foresee that you would stay there on a permanent basis. It is a solution until you were able to get better and then you could go. If you need long-term care it would be within your unit.

I guess the nursing facilities that I visited, and I don't want it to sound like a copout, but it's just, they're awful. You walk in and everything's the seventies green. It's all very institutional.

J. Hoadley. My particular expertise is in nursing home and intergenerational day care centers. I don't believe that nursing homes are to be on the back 10 acres of a 50 acre site. I don't believe it's true. I like it integrated right in there, it's exactly where it should be. It should be right where downtown is or most of the mobility. If they can't go to the downtown, it would be really neat if they could see it there. But you say you don't want to, so I think that's a pretty important thing that we need to look at. These projects really are urban designs, they're really group planning problems. You're designing for one segment of a community and all of the projects are trying to get the community into the project, yet we're beginning to see a sort of fear to draw the community into it. Both of the projects have the downtown in the right location. I would like to see what's on the other side of the property line and how you can draw those folks in. We as architects pick a drawing scale that equals the site but, I think that your project would be supported by saying: "There's an awful lot of people living right south of there and down here by the duplex plug, and over here by this other drawing that could be drawn into this center." We shouldn't have a fear of providing a complete range of services in a CCRC. Don't be afraid to design it.

K. Brandle. You didn't make a little bit larger a plan of the community around. I'm living just about two blocks away from the site you are using. To the west of this whole site there is a very large group of recent larger town-house, condominium-type rental housing. These people who live there would like to be in a community center like you planned there. They would love that because particularly you will have a lot of customers. This road is a very important road. It's much stronger than you actually show it there, because it swings all the way around and connects with the rest of the neighborhood. So there would be a tremendous spill-over and this could be a real center, not at the edge as we see it now and not just an entry to the retirement community. What I wonder about is why are people interested in living there? Why would they go? I feel that when we design something like this we try to duplicate our American one-family house. And I'm not so sure that all people think like this when they come to that age where they get in a frame of mind that "I have another 20 years or whatever, maybe I should live in another situation." Naturally the Europeans have a very different situation because they don't have the land and most of them live in apartments. But because you want to have that security you really like to live close to other people. You still would like to have privacy, but you want to be closer because if something happens you can call for help. If you design the same thing that we have now it will be a bedroom community in a sense with even less activity. Because people aren't working anymore. I'm not so sure that for that group of people something like this would fly. You see there is not enough activity here.

G. Tipton. I'd like to talk about your research. What did you find to be the range of ages that people would move to a retirement community? In some ways what you've created there is pretty much the same as the typical retirement community with a little less emphasis on nursing and more emphasis, perhaps, on a commercial maybe linked to the neighborhood. Then you introduced the notion of the 50-60 year olds.

Madelyn. The 50-60 year olds are a starting age.

G. Tipton. The average entry age of residents in a continuing care retirement community in this country is 75 years and over. Whereas the cul-de-sac housing might appeal to a younger segment. There's 25 years age difference between a 50-year old and a 75-year old. Several projects that we've been exploring right now are looking at the possibility of co-mingling that younger age population. Why would they choose to move there? What services are provided to the younger elderly that would be desirable versus the older elderly? In this country at least, and maybe it's just the way it's been over the years, we have this emphasis on compartmentalizing ourselves into a group that we belong to. We feel a little bit uncomfortable moving to this segment because we don't belong in that group. Let's say, I'm 55, I'm 60 years old, I don't belong in this retirement community. And those people who move into independent living say "Well, I'm not an assisted living person."

D. Cinelli. Well, I thought you were talking about yourself. I'd say you look great for 55.

G. Tipton. It's been tough. Architecture is a tough profession. Anybody who is about to graduate should know that we're aging fast, so we're well suited to doing retirement communities. But that's an issue, the broader definition of a retirement community, who it appeals to and why they choose to live there.

D. Cinelli. If the site plan was an exercise to get to the bigger picture that you've thrown up for us to look at, I think that you've really hurt yourself on the master plan by not really paying attention to some significant graphics, the things that make a difference. They are really there but I can't see them. I mean the walking paths are of the same tone as the car. I think you've gone through this whole exercise to be able to make the separation. You say that this is a community but you don't tell me what's in there. As far as I'm concerned, this road here could be off any road. I mean it could be off this road here. You could have said: "What I'm focussing on is doing a sub-development of 20 units on a typical suburban street and this thing is really an out-placement from a hospital that's down the street that provides home health care when this person wants their blood pressure taken." The thing that bothers me about it is that the biggest pigeon that you've thrown up for me to focus on is this development here. Now you've told me that you're going to keep somebody in here as long as they possibly can to age in place. So you're dealing with walkers, you're dealing with wheelchairs, you've gone through this whole exercise and appear to understand the major problems. And I start to look at this and I say: "This is a single family house." You don't have the 1'6" needed to the left side of the door to be able to get at the door and open it. The tub, the water closet in such a place where it's difficult to transfer. How do I age in place in this facility? I really don't think you've addressed a lot of the issues of aging in place. But, you've given me this as the biggest target to look at. I think that if you want somebody to age in place and live there as long as they possibly can, then you have really got to get into the micro-environment and say: "I'm doing something different that the builder down the street is not doing. I'm making empty nester housing for a person who is 60 years old who is going to move in here and be able to live here as long as he possibly can because of this and this and this." I think you need to spend a lot more time on developing that.

G. Tipton. Was that your concept, that that would be the place that one lived and aged in place and not move progressively to other parts of this community (Figure 7.4)?

Madelyn. Yes.

G. Tipton. I agree with Dan, I kind of struggled to see where was pedestrian and where was auto. In some ways it does follow the traditional planning techniques used to organize retirement communities with pedestrian ways to a community center separated from cars. What Dan also pointed out are some of the traditional things that we look for almost instinctively when we design for aging in

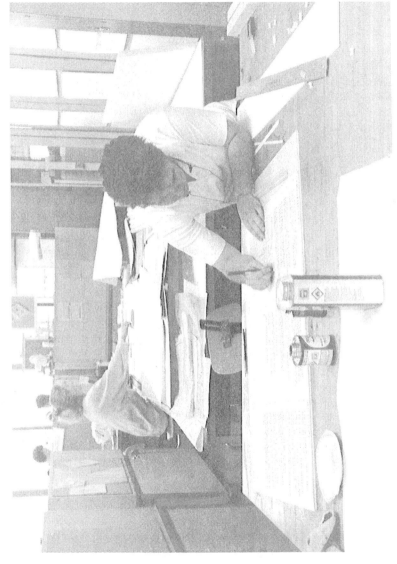

FIGURE 7.4. Working Toward the Design Jury

place. The access for a wheelchair or walker and other details which
perhaps time didn't permit you to get into.

N. Levine. What we're really saying today is a retirement community. We can take the word retirement or the program for a
retirement community off the hook. What we're really asking ourselves is: at what age do we begin to address planning for retirement? Basically what you're looking at over there is a two bedroom
single family type of structure. To get into the infrastructure and say
that there's 18" needed next to the door knob and things like that,
that's moot at this stage of the game because the attempt is to find
out the behavioral context of how does man want to live and address his environment. She's looked at the front porch over there
and she's saying: "That's a possibility for a person who comes out
in the morning." She's saying that maybe the older person who
comes out and reads the newspaper might see his neighbor and take
a walk down to the community center. Not having that little porch
would mean the person stayed back in their bed over there half the
day and passed eating breakfast. We're looking at: how do we grow
old within the context of that development? We go back to the site
and say: "If we pick up all of the constraints that the site has to
offer us, at what age would I want to live within the context of that
sort of environment?" You could say that we've got a nice little
courtyard, we have options as far as the passive environment and a
semi-public environment, a semi-private type of environment. Now
if we want to take the title away it's a heck of a community and you
just have to say, how old would you want to be to really move here.
For all practical purposes what we're saying is that as we're designing and thinking of what we're doing for the future as far as how we
age, we should start at a much younger age, because that community is no different than where you would like to live right now. Those
offerings are there for your options to select them. The community
center wants to react to the aged individual. It has a nutritional
program, a possible PT program, a possible OT program, as far as
therapies are concerned, but that also can be a spa for the center of a
major community; and if you change the terminology and the jar-
gon you'd get to find out what motivates an individual. To quote a
great fan who said that our environment has a language to offer us
and how we deal with that language motivates us as an individual to

be able to act and interact within the context of our own lifestyle. If you make it that easy to respond to, it can serve all ages. For example, if you have lakes, you're going to have a person who wants to sit and watch the water and watch a bird or a duck playing with that. Or you can have an individual who says, I don't like the water, I've got trees to look out onto. You know the younger individual that says, I can take a walk into town and do my workout. As you offer all those choices, you have now activated a community which has a life to offer and life is what we're really talking about, life-style, no matter at what age.

As far as the physical structure, there's so many things coming into the marketplace today. Even as a practicing professional it is difficult to keep up with it. We're going to have to include it whether we like it or not. Whether it's a grab bar, the space between the door knob and the wall–and there are other factors as far as ramps and stairs and what have you–but most important is that you're learning what we should do now, so that we as human beings understand what we're dealing with.

The problem is that you've got that many acres for only 375 units. I could tell you bluntly and unequivocally it cannot support it economically. It's an impossibility to pull it off and have that much there. It would have to have something far more dense and especially with the ecology of the site and all the constraints you're dealing with. It's a tough site economically. So you have to build the broader picture. I can support this and get into the understanding of the process of aging as an area program that you want to address. But I think that all the single family housing to the west and what you've got to the south is all a part of this because it's too small to stand on its own feet.

D. Cinelli. The problem I have is that what she's looking at is an urban fabric, an urban typology, and then a suburban typology and rural typology. I'd like to see this as a six-unit assisted living building. And I'd like to be able to see a lot, within the confines of this suburban-looking vernacular, so that if I no longer can take care of myself here, and I can't have home health care addressed to me any more because it becomes too expensive, I can still live within this neighborhood. I think that a lot of suburban areas can deal with a micro CCRC versus always having to deal with CCRCs that are 350-500 unit involvements.

J. Turner. A couple of questions that I want to raise. The first question is, in starting the project did you first attempt to develop a profile of the mix and the density, a general description of what you wanted this retirement community to be?

Madelyn. When I first started I covered the whole site pretty much with single family housing. It was very dense. Then I backed off and concentrated more on the community development because it was an important key to the rest of the surrounding area. I tried to figure out what services, and how that relates back out. And then I started looking at this area here, the micro, not the unit itself, but the community type of situation.

J. Turner. As you found yourself getting into that process did some campuses emerge where you began to establish desired mixes of the go-goes and the no-goes, or the more dependent elderly to the more active elderly? Did you try to develop some percentages or numbers of how many units from each kind will be on the site?

Madelyn. No, I didn't.

J. Turner. As a developer who works with site planners I have to convince my banker of the justification of this program. Therefore I'm always asking the question why. Why this development in this location? Why should these prospective residents relocate in this environment? And underlying all of that is, what is the economic justification? Does this have a value for the resident or it won't be successful. And my observation would be for those of you who are devoting your careers to this that you're an observer, a viewer. You may or may not have a lot of experience in senior housing. You would probably be benefited greatly if you could share your knowledge initially by defining the program, by profiling the mix, the density, the interrelationship of the mix, so that you could quickly determine what the overall capacity of the site is and what is the overall relationship of the uses. The viewer cannot get into a lot of the architectural details in the site plan without it. Through both of the presentations I have been grappling with questions such as: is there really a skilled care facility as a part of these two plans or isn't there, I think that what I'm hearing is that there isn't. My recommendation would be that early on you should bullet and profile some of the more key elements of the plan. If you don't believe that skilled care is a significant part of the plan, then you should highlight that for your jury and then you can offer justification as to why (Figure 7.5).

R. Sekulski. Not being an architect, my vision of the process of design is probably quite a bit different than most people here. I understand and see your presentation as a planned view of facilities but I really wonder if you were to approach a design problem from the user perspective, from the height, from the location, from the sense and feel of an elderly person. What is that environment to me, having limited capabilities. How would I create adjacencies and relationships with my peers, my cohorts, and then the proximity of spaces, adjacencies, functional buildings and so on? I see the presentations and I think that this is the way we present as architects. This is how we think of space and relationships. But sometimes it's good to think differently and then shake up your concept. It can give you a whole different perspective and a new vision.

T. Hille. I have a comment on the cul-de-sac that is jumping out at me. And I think it's something that applies to all of the conditions that you're setting up here. It seems to me that you're putting a really high priority on the unit of that size. That's really important to you and I think the reason you're doing that is because it's mostly social interaction. Your idea there is that I don't have a back garden, let's say, you have a view out to an untouched landscape. Is that it? On the cul-de-sac? What is on the back side of these houses?

Madelyn. On this side is the view of the lake. People like to sit there. And this side can be green, like a park area in the back.

T. Hille. If you look at the way a small town in the midwest is traditionally laid out, you would have a backyard. Let's say that you don't need much of a backyard because that's just a maintenance problem. But you would normally have that in a block situation in a small town and you would have a rear neighbor as well as front neighbors and that's another opportunity for social interaction that in your case you're missing. You opt for a kind of pristine view to the landscape which is another idea, but ultimately the pristine to the landscape is, I think, a little muddy, because you have an almost urban scheme at the same time with the row houses. So, I worry that, maybe, you end up with the worst of both worlds. That you

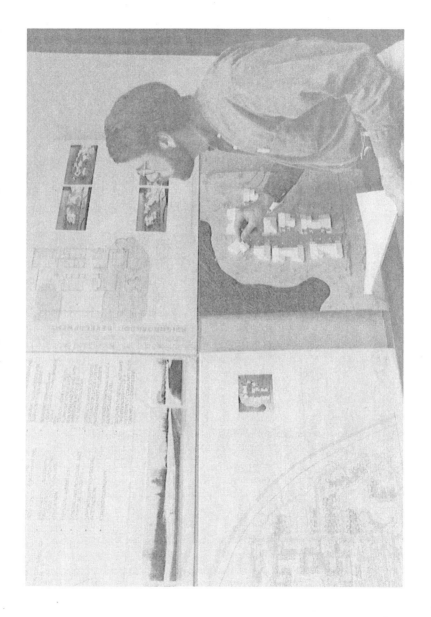

FIGURE 7.5. A Jury Member Reviews the Project

have this kind of density that you would get in an urban context where you would have a lot of contact and a lot of different dimensions. You can have front neighbors, back neighbors, side neighbors, all kinds of neighbors, but you don't get much landscape, it's an urban context. Or you can have a house in the country where you get a lot of landscaping and no neighbors. And you're trying to work somewhere in between and I find that the units you're setting seem to be a bit too isolated for me. One dimension it's social, on the other dimension it related to the landscape as well. For instance, the corner off the lake, if you eliminated the two units right at the corner, the one that's at the angle and the one below it, your public space that you're setting up in your cul-de-sac street begins to actually relate to the lake. But you don't offer that. It's completely compartmentalized, so it becomes too internal, I think.

I would also think in terms of this front and back garden. Gardening seems a positive thing to at least offer as an option. Is this is a small garden space in front? That would make a nice flower garden, maybe, not such a great vegetable garden. Could you have a vegetable garden? Is there a way you could begin to claim that here?

Madelyn. Off the back.

T. Hille. Depending on whether that's the front side of the unit to the south or whether that's to the north. Does that take advantage of the sun? For instance if I have the front porch that catches south light versus the porch that faces the north for nine months out of the year. To me that standardization should be reconsidered to at least offer the option of sitting in private versus sitting in public, or sitting in the sun versus sitting in the shade.

H. Naimark. I am 67 and still the go-go generation and I was trying to think why this would appeal to us. I think the motivation would be that it is related to the University and we could take advantage of all those activities in the University very easily both coming and going. I also think that most of us think that one of us is going to be alone one day. And the nice part about moving into a community like this is that you feel that when one goes the other one has developed a circle of friends which I think is extremely important. The appeal of having all these services here is central. Most people have to really search here and search there and search every other place for services. Even the things you've talked about, health care and health related support services, house cleaning, shopping. I think those services have to be accessible or at least be thought of. How do you get the groceries from the store back to your house, if you don't want to drive any more? So, I think the appeal really is that it's in the University setting, and I think a small single home in this kind of a community is what I would see as the ideal for someone like me. We're both college educated and I think that the environment would just be terrific. I think that's the appeal. I also would like to take out the word "retirement." As soon as I see "retirement community" I want to run. I think we have to find a new name that does not classify and stereotype people.

The last component that I would like to see in there is offering some of that for students, live-ins. We try to have younger friends. Unfortunately our equals are dying. We try to have younger friends because, first of all, they're very stimulating and they don't talk about their aches and pains. Certainly it would be an ideal place for students to live in. I think they would create that intergenerational concept so that people would feel that they're not moving in with older people. It would really add a component that would make it very attractive.

G. Tipton. I think that's pretty much what most people who are seeking a vital retirement are looking for. They use the word continuum of care as closely to the style of living they're used to but that range of services all the way up through.

H. Naimark. I think there should be continuum of care. I agree with you. So that you're not moving out of the community, when you eventually need to have higher skilled care.

G. Tipton. The nursing home has truly gotten a bad rap over the years. There's really a lot of environmental design research that's needed for this environment. There's some creative direction going on today, but a lot more is needed. I'd just like to make a couple of quick observations. When Ben called me and asked me to participate in the jury today, one of the things that I was hoping was actually to learn something through the process as well as to add to it if I could. I kind of came accepting the fact that there would be grossly wrong programmatic relationships between the amount of community space and the amount of units. I shouldn't judge the academic world, to say that, okay, that's left to the real world to learn about. Forgive me for saying that. What I was hoping for, though, was an exploration of areas that the real world doesn't sometimes allow us to do. I was hoping that the design of the residential unit was going to be tackled here in this particular one through some really in-depth look-see at what aging in place is all about and how it might be resolved.

L. Pastalan. You haven't seen them all yet.

G. Tipton. I'm sorry, but perhaps the cul-de-sac and then the unit have been somewhat of an emphasis here. The resolution of the living space is pretty much as we've seen before and still doesn't resolve many of the aging in place issues. It was my hope that I was going to see something new and fresh. New explorations, something that in fact could take back a new perspective on that. The only reason I'm bringing that point up is because you said that you were emphasizing the residential side. It really boiled down to that social model what that cul-de-sac was all about as opposed to the living unit itself, I think. It's just an observation.

L. Pastalan. If I may, I'd like to ask Bob Foreman who is the Director of Alumni Relations at The University of Michigan. Why would somebody who's currently living in Florida, California, or Arizona or wherever want to come back and take part in this kind of community?

B. Foreman. That's a good question, Lee. I've been sitting here trying to think of something bright and qualified to say. My only expertise is dealing with the alumni. I see it at all ages and all stages of their lives. I don't think alumni come back to Ann Arbor to recapture the fountain of youth or even to relive their halcyon days. We do have a great many alumni/alumnae who come back to Ann Arbor choosing whatever housing is available, and frequently trying to get in close physical proximity to the campus, because there are lots of things going on there that are exciting to them. So they want to go to basketball games and theater and take advantage. They're not really trying to relive something as much as they're trying to do what they should have, or wanted to do when they were students and there was no time to do it. They're entering a very exciting part of their own lives where they're freer to do some of the things they've always wished to do and they wish to do it in a university community as opposed to country club.

We've brought in the Alumni Association a whole series of continuing education programs for Alumni/Alumnae on campus in our Alumni Center for people who come some distance all within an hour's drive. Because they're intellectually stimulated by the kinds of things we're offering. When I see these kinds of facilities I get excited because I'd like to export some of our programming on site around here. This means not only what's being done with our faculty, but what's being done with our student alumni. Actually we've got some programs there and people are eager to be involved in this kind of activity. So, I don't get excited from my point of view as to what any of these environments have or don't have. The proximity to the institution is a major plus and the people are coming back for that. Now, for every person who comes back, there is that person who wishes to do deep sea fishing or golfing. I find this an interesting exercise to begin to think about in terms of my own life, and I don't know if we plan as well as we ought to. I like this idea of aging in place. We've suddenly become very, very serious about aging in place, but most of us don't think about it in those terms. We don't simply think about what's our lifestyle going to be like? What are the things that would excite us? This has become very much a place where alumni/alumnae wish to come back for a whole variety of reasons. Many of them don't come and stay 12 months. They come back and live for part of the year. These, again, are educated people who are reasonably active and they look at themselves and in many cases have not reached the point where they're seriously considering what their health care needs are going to be and their nursing care and what have you, but they have a kind of image that the University with all its medical facilities, all those kinds of outreach programs, will take care of them. How that's going to happen in reality is something else. So, yes they come back in, I think, sizeable numbers to try to be intellectually stimulated and I think in general they are. And they'll live all over the place.

D. Cinelli. A comment about CCRCs in general as I see them in the future. What we see is that the Marriott and the Corporations that are doing these communities have a ratio on zoning and financing these deals in about 1 in 20. I think that these are the numbers that someone was telling me in terms of going in and getting a 50 acre parcel and trying to get it zoned. You can spend a million dollars trying to get it zoned and then at the end not having it being done. There are a number of projects that you can buy from the Resolution Trust right now because of default. Bankers and financing experts look at these mega deals harder and harder all the time.

I think that what you will see in the future is less of the big projects and a lot more of these. A lot of the hospitals that got involved with retirement communities have no business doing them, because they don't understand the development business for the most part. What hospitals and health care environments are going to want to do is what they do well. They may deliver health care within the homes or deliver care into the health care institutions. So my sense is that you're going to see more and more smaller CCRCs, micro communities where it's easier to get it zoned, where it's easier to get it financed. Health care providers will be able to take the health care portion of their communities. When someone is moving into a retirement community, what they're doing for the most part is trying to take whatever life-style they had living before in this single family house and drag it with them into this other environment. And as they age in place they no longer can get to the store, they no longer can get to other services, they want to be able to have those things be provided to them. My sense is that unless the Japanese are going to continue to finance some of these things the big CCRCs are really a wave of the past.

G. Tipton. Another point of view. From my experience what's happening in CCRCs is going in both directions. More and more people are looking for ways to do smaller facilities because of all the reasons you've put forth. Certainly if you could integrate this into the infrastructure like a university setting that has a lot of things already going for it, it's great. It makes an awful lot of sense because otherwise it kind of sets itself in a corn-field. Then you run into the financial realities, you can't afford to support with 20 units all the services you want to bring. So the integration makes an awful lot of sense. The other thing is that there are retirement communities that have a vitality in and of themselves. If you can overlap that with the vitality that already exists with a university setting, I think you've got a dynamite situation going. Usually the reason the bigger ones are gravitated towards other places is to create the vitality that's really needed to make it a good place to be. I think that for these communities to succeed they have got to be an integral part of a vital community to start with, not plunked down in a corn-field. That's just an observation. I think it's going in both directions right now. Fewer people are doing the big ones. That's for sure.

Madelyn. Thank you.

Hierarchy of Needs

Michael Nicklowitz
Kwang-Sun Choi

Kwang-Sun. First of all we are going to explain our concept. Based on Maslow's Hierarchy of Needs there are five human needs reflecting constant motivations. They are: (1) *Physiological needs,* such as food, water, sex and shelter; (2) *Safety needs,* relating to protection against external danger or threat, be it deprivation, or personal security; (3) *Social needs,* such as the giving and receiving of love, friendship, affection, belonging, association, and acceptance; (4) *Ego needs* of two types–the need for autonomy and independence as well as the need for self-esteem and self-worth, derived from status, recognition, appreciation and so forth; and (5) *Self-actualization needs,* including the need to achieve one's potential or the need for ongoing self-development (Figure 8.1).

Throughout our design phase we constantly referred to Maslow's hierarchy. But in the middle of the session, we found that architecture can provide the needs only up to a certain level. Architects can provide the physiological needs and the environmental needs. The social and psychological needs have to be provided by others and the psychological needs maybe are provided by the person him/herself. We used color coding in our plans to present the different needs.

The other thing we focused on was the concept of aging in place. One of the ladies here mentioned that retirement in Western cultures does not enjoy high status. But in my country, Korea, retirement is

[Haworth co-indexing entry note]: "Hierarchy of Needs." Nicklowitz, Michael, and Kwang-Sun Choi. Co-published simultaneously in *Journal of Housing for the Elderly* (The Haworth Press, Inc.) Vol. 11, No. 1, 1994, pp. 121-143; and: *University-Linked Retirement Communities: Student Visions of Eldercare* (ed: Leon A. Pastalan, and Benyamin Schwarz) The Haworth Press, Inc., 1994, pp. 121-143. Multiple copies of this article/chapter may be purchased from The Haworth Document Delivery Center [1-800-3-HAWORTH; 9:00 a.m. - 5:00 p.m. (EST)].

FIGURE 8.1. Maslow's Hierarchy of Needs

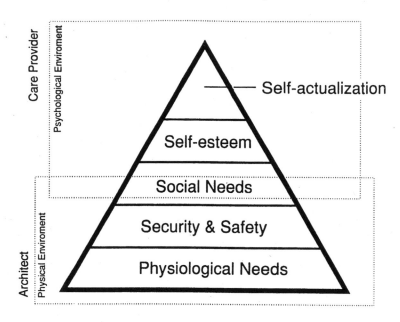

something different. Old person means something very good. You are more respectable, more a kind of new stage in your life. Aging starts from the birth, not from 60 or 65 or 70. Aging starts from birth and continues throughout life, and that is a very important concept.

Michael. Okay, we'll start from these two concepts. What this diagram shows is that there's a real interaction between the residents and the present faculty (Figure 8.2). I mean the faculty can look at the residents as a resource and they can tap into that resource. And at the same time the residents have a sense of belonging, providing that the faculty views its role in typical educational terms where the faculty provides that service to the students and the students tap into the faculty as a resource. But most importantly what I see really helping this project along would be these relationships where the student body can now be a resource for the residents. It may work out that some of the nursing students or others become heavily involved in how this complex is facilitated, and at

FIGURE 8.2. The Interaction Diagram

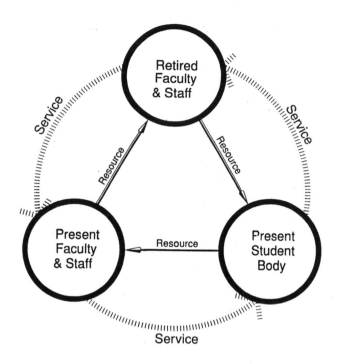

the same time the residents become a resource for the nursing students and the nursing students become caregivers.

Figure 8.3 describes our thinking process through the development of a floor plan. Initially we started out with a typical nursing home plan and we worked our way through these different floor plans studying a lot of the Scandinavian style nursing homes. Slowly we worked our way into this courtyard scene. One important thing that we had found out that's a little bit different between the Scandinavian culture and our culture is the use of the car. The car is such a personal thing to Americans, where in that culture it's just a real luxury for people to have because of the cost of the car, the cost of fuel and taxes and so forth. We asked ourselves: "What do we do? How do we integrate cars in this Scandinavian way of thinking into our site?"

If we move over to the site plan we have here the main entry

FIGURE 8.3. A Representation of the Thinking Process

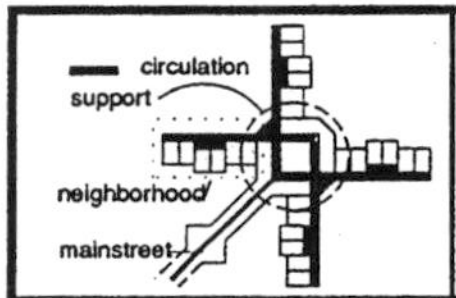	Originally the plan began to emulate a standard Nursing Care Center plan with single loaded corridors radiating from a central support core. This plan was some what so-	cially stagnant and extremely rigid in form, lending itself more to the function of the care giver and less to the comfort of the resident.
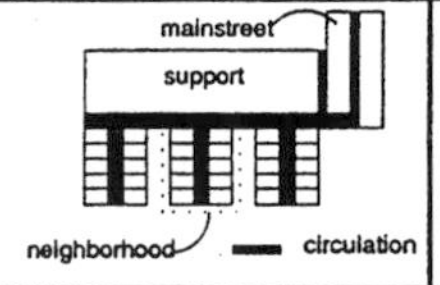	Clustering the dwelling units into a double loaded corridor arrangement began to set up a some what forced social petal setting with neighbors along the corridor while the	backyards became close together infringing on the private zones. The organization of neighborhood support areas and Main Street activity areas lacked order.
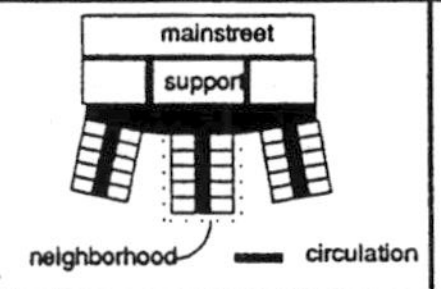	By stacking the Main Street activity area beyond the neighborhood support areas next to the neighborhoods, a sense of order becomes clearer. (As you move closer to Main Street the levels of activity become greater.) Radiating the	neighborhoods around the center, backyards are separated to a greater extent, however the negative is that they still open up at the ends to public areas.
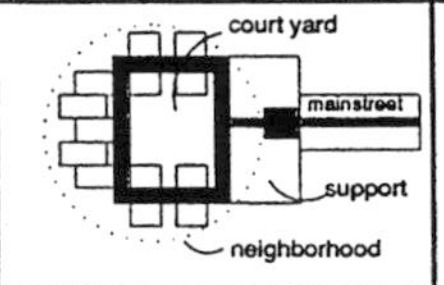	Providing a circulation loop will capture a courtyard which can be shared by the neighborhood. This semi-private space provides a socialization area, however this arrange-	ment becomes violated by placing some dwelling units within the courtyard.
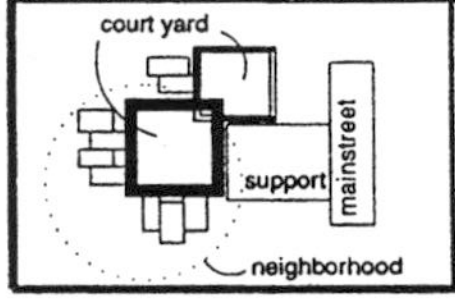	Placing dwelling units around the perimeter of the courtyard helped the plan accomplish several positive aspects. • A social petal arrangement (not forced) around the semi-private courtyard. • An organized layering of privacy from semi-private drives to private backyards and dwelling units to semi-	private front porch and protected walkway to a semi-public neighborhood support area to a public Main Street area. (A sense of retreat and an encouragement for socialization becomes an easy choice.) • Overlapping courtyards produce interesting transitions from dwelling units to neighborhood support areas.

point from Green Road (Figure 8.4). Then we have what we're calling a Main Street facility which is basically this whole diagonal axis through the center of the complex. And then working our way out we have cluster housing which is essentially condominium style living that is all worked in around these internal courtyards. And then at the end of Main Street we have, as another alternative style of living, a mid-rise apartment style. We understood that the cost of living in these cluster homes is going to be high. We're aiming it towards past faculty and staff at the University so they're educated people, hopefully at the higher end of middle income. Maybe lower end of upper income so they can afford this. So anyway, what I'm saying is that we just provided an alternative to the mid-rise building.

The concepts that we had here is that we're progressing through these different levels of activity that are building up to Main Street. Over here we have a more subdued environment and you work your way into neighborhood gatherings which pretty much service the surrounding cluster housing complex. The type of amenities that we have here are things like a bakery, hospitality suite for parties, etc. It might be for somebody who lives in this complex that is giving a birthday party and they can rent this little hall and have a private party in there for them, bar, lounge. We felt it was important that, instead of clumping administration into one large area anywhere in this complex, it will be better to spread it out and disperse it. We have a greenhouse over here. There are seven units that pretty much surround the courtyard, and potentially there may be plots of land that people may want to get into gardening. They can start some things in the greenhouse in the winter and come out and plant them in here (Figure 8.5).

Basically what we're thinking is that we'll provide the socialization here. What is unique about our design is that we have these complete networks of covered walkways so that people don't really have to go outside to get to Main Street. They can go as far to an activity area as they want without leaving the complex, so it becomes a little more useful year round. We have this corridor set up with resting and small socialization areas. You've got to give elderly people a spot to stop. We don't want it to look like a resting spot. We want it to look like a normal thing where they sit down and visit.

FIGURE 8.4. Site Plan

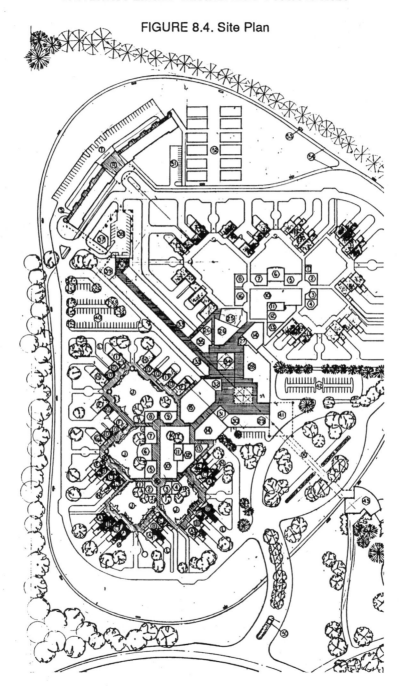

Site Plan Legend

Cluster Housing: Single Story

A   One Bedroom
B   One Bedroom with a Den/1
C   One Bedroom with a Den/2
D   Two Bedroom - Garage Conv.
E   Two Bedroom

Cluster Housing: Stacked Units

F   One Bedroom with a Den/1
G   One Bedroom with a Den/2
H   Two Bedroom
I   Two Bedroom with a Den

Neighborhood Facilities

1   Bakery
2   Hospitality Suite
3   Bar / Lounge
4   Administration
5   Activity Room
6   Greenhouse
7   Game Room
8   Administration
9   Beauty Salon
10 Neighborhood Commons
11 Security / Med-Alert
12 Kitchen
13 Laundry
14 Mechanical / Shop
15 Exercise / Squash / Pool
16 Wood Shop

Cluster Housing: General

J   Neighborhood Courtyard
K   Enclosed Walkways
L   Private Driveway
M   Primary Entry
O   Shared Garage

Mid-Rise Housing

P   One Bedroom
Q   Two Bedroom
R   Commons
S   Lower Level Garage
T   Guest Parking

Main Street Facilities

25 Movie Theater
26 Medical Clinics
27 Ice Cream Parlor
28 Day Care Intergener
29 Office
30 Grocery/Drug Store
31 Bank
32 Post Office
33 Retail Shops
34 Worship Area
35 Library
36 North Lobby Main Street
37 Vertical Core of Offices
38 Office Building Parking
39 North Entry Main Street
40 Community Parking
41 South Entry Main Street
42 Admin. / Parking
43 Family Restaurant
44 Restaurant Parking
45 Pedestrian Bridge
46 Wolverine Lake
50 Sentry
51 Electrical Cart Parking
52 Tennis Courts
53 Bench Seating
54 Cart and Walking Path

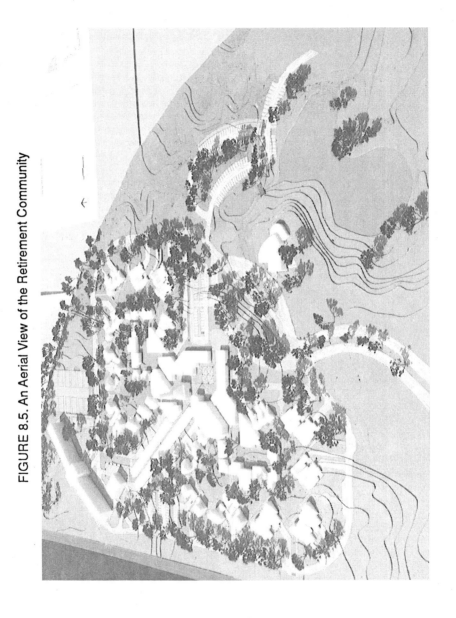

FIGURE 8.5. An Aerial View of the Retirement Community

It becomes an uncomfortable thing for an older person to walk too many paces and start breathing real heavy and lean on a handrail or something. We want it to be a natural thing so that they will have a way to progress through this site at their own pace.

Main Street becomes a resource for the outside community. We picture this as being maybe a large scale Nickels Arcade or small mall type of environment where there is some interaction between outsiders and the people who live here. In fact, we've allocated some of this Main Street to shops and offices that may be run by the residents themselves. So what's happening here is that people who are aging now have a purpose. They have a shop here that they run and that they can tie into the community through what they're doing in the shop. It's a kind of continuing program through their career. In actuality they are not retiring. This is an alternative lifestyle.

An important part of this site are these medical centers. We're calling them MedAlert. This is how the service is now being provided to all the residents. There can be passive monitoring systems there to keep track of people who are in need of more services. Passively means where it doesn't become too intrusive to their lifestyle. For example, in one Scandinavian project that we studied where they had Alzheimer's patients who were free to move about, not only the community but outside the community into the city. And the way that they were monitored was that electronic bracelet on the wrist. So when it became time to eat or whatever and they didn't come back the monitors knew where they were and they could go get them and bring them back.

We have here a physical therapy, or an exercise area. It might have squash courts, spas and a swimming pool. We also incorporated a post office and a grocery store within the complex which we felt was important. At the main entrance of Main Street we have what we're calling an intergenerational day-care center. This becomes a drop-off area for kids and adults and it may be used by the residents, but more probably, by the outside community. It becomes another draw to bring the outside community into the complex. We have a medical clinic and a movie house as part of Main Street. On the other side you have the other neighborhood which is designed with a semi-public space and then back into a private dwelling place. Here we have outside tennis courts.

We hope to draw in not only the people who are 65,75 on up. We want to start this at least at 50 if not sooner to get that mix that we feel is important. Looking as we go down Main Street, this actually has a connector link as the second level which brings you into the mid-rise. One thing I left out is there's a satellite restaurant on the site by this man-made lake. This is just another draw for the community. People who live here might want to meet with somebody not in their semi-public dining facility, but maybe in a full fledged restaurant. Then there's the mid-rise here which is for up to 200 residents. About 100 residents are spread out through the cluster housing.

Kwang-Sun. We studied some European models. In Korea we have similar retirement communities but they are a little bit different. There is one big community that we call a retired artists village. The persons who live there have a kind of sense of belonging. We were hoping to create this sense of belonging by providing this environment for retired faculty and alumni.

I wanted to say another thing. Frankly speaking, this is the first time for me to design an American style home. I have designed apartments, office buildings, or schools. I think that homes are quite different. I found this very difficult. I changed this floor plan many times. Ben gave me a lot of thoughts. He asked: why the living room had to be here ? What was the relationship to the corridor? Why bedrooms should open to the corridor? In my country you don't have these problems. Because the living room should always face the entrance. It's kind of communal. In Korea we don't have privacy in the same sense as in this culture. We don't have the term "mine." Instead we have just "ours." Even in our language we don't say "my wife." We say "our wife." So the concept of privacy is very difficult. "Our wife" means that she's my wife as well as my mother's daughter-in-law, and my daughter's mother; the term "wife" has many connotations.

So for three or four weeks I struggled to design these one bedroom and two bedroom type units. I reviewed the literature about aging and environment. It was very hard for me. As you can see we didn't develop a full design, we just developed an idea, a concept. Here is the typical floor plan. You can see the small junctions that can provide a place for the social needs. I mean people will be able to come, and just sit here and talk. In the center of each floor we provided a kitchen where they will come and have their breakfast together. We provided a patio in every central place so that the residents will come together and be able to enjoy the outside.

These mid-rise apartments are designed for the persons who are not able to move into these single family houses. The apartments are much smaller than the cottage type. The residents should be able to use the main streets. We don't want to isolate them from the whole project.

G. Tipton. Excuse me, are those programmatic elements in the mid-rise similar in ways to the other housing?

Michael. Yes.

G. Tipton. Providing similar functions and uses?

Michael. Right. Very similar. What I did here is I blew up an 1/8″ small scale of these single story clustered homes and what you're looking at here is the internal courtyard (Figure 8.6). These are the doorways into that courtyard and then the covered walkway which is this terra cotta color. That is the network that you've seen through this whole complex.

G. Tipton. Covered and enclosed?

Michael. Covered and enclosed. What could happen in three months out of the year is that, maybe they could open some of these up and it becomes more of an outdoor space. We felt that it is important that this space will feel as though you're in a courtyard. So it's basically an all glass wall unit. In these corners you have the socialization areas which would diffuse the light and become a way finding device different from the hallway. It reminds you where you are. Another thought was also taking care of the light issue that you have at the end of the long hallway. This can prevent the glare on the floor.

In the units themselves you can have guests come over. You have a back patio. A gated landscaped patio. A living area. We thought that it was an important aspect to be able to have guests over. So we provided in here a foldout bed. You have a laundry area so that you shouldn't have to go out and do your laundry in the center. Here are the bedrooms with outdoor views. This is important because if at some point one may become bedridden for a long period of time one should be able to have contact with the outdoors. The window-

FIGURE 8.6. A Floor Plan of a Housing Cluster

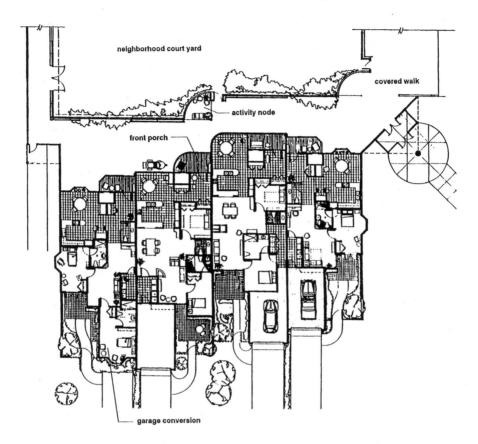

sills are low enough that you should be able to see outside as you're lying in bed. Large bathrooms. Maybe this is just a large bathroom here, but as you progress down it becomes equipped with grab bars and so forth. And up at the front end of the unit that faces the courtyard you have a large kitchen with a lot of counter space. The idea there is to keep much of the cabinetry work down lower and accessible for those who may be in a wheelchair. And another thing that we see happening in a lot of Scandinavian designs is that they had adjustable counters which is such a great idea. I don't understand why they don't use that more here so that you can adjust it to give a small woman the flexibility. She might not want the counter the same height as an elderly man or a young man living right next door. So there's that flexibility while she gets things where she wants them. They're comfortable.

The front porch, which is another place for socialization area, can have neighbors over and you can see people walking through this walkway. This is to maintain the contact with the outside world. This is a bedroom or a den that could actually function as a bedroom so that if you want somebody to move in with you temporarily or if you want guests over, they've got more private setting here. This unit is 1100 square feet and this one here is about 1300 square feet. Basically they're all set up the same. In this unit there is somebody who doesn't drive a car any more, yet she wants to keep her sphere of activity as large as she can. So this network will accommodate electrical carts.

I was working on a project in Adrian for Sister Catherine, Catholic sisters. They have major headquarters out there. They have some network of links between the buildings. These are tunnels that connect all these different facilities and they can literally ride around on these carts. They'll get out from where they live and they'll go down and around to the kitchen and get breakfast and they'll go down and around to where they work. And it's amazing. I saw a chart in there that showed the profile of the age of these people who live there. It went from 50 to 60 to 80 to 90 to 100. They have people who were 100 years old, and many of these people are still working. They go off to work and they function and produce work for the community. And that's the idea that I had here with that network and the idea of Main Street. Eventually when somebody becomes bedridden, they have more services provided to them. They don't have to get up and move to a nursing home.

Also there may come a time when the garage is no longer a useful space so I thought, why not convert that to another bedroom. We have these exterior walls. And maybe a relative or a student can come and live here. There's the idea of human resource where a student can get the incentive of free housing if he or she takes care of an Alzheimer's patient for eight hours out of the day.

D. Cinelli. Or a live-in nurse.

Michael. So, I guess what I'm trying to do is to show you the progression of how the apartment adapts. There are building features like oxygen nooks. We have TV in the bedroom which could be also a cable network system that ties into the University channel that keeps people close. Even though they're in bed they can get that link to the outdoors to see what's going on. The computer network we thought was important, you see that in the floor plan. A type of mechanical system that is suitable for elderly. Safe appliances. We've talked about it and planned for it so that these things are set up in a way where, if this was your oven and this was your counter, it's important to keep them level. Your oven door should maybe line up with the counter. So that when you drag out something hot and you're in a wheelchair it should make it an easy transition. And the idea of bolting down appliances because accidents can happen. An individual mailbox adds to that individuality where if you have a mailman that comes by and drops mail in your box it's a little bit more personal. There are two toilet rooms in the unit. We felt that it's something important because a person who is in a wheelchair needs the bathroom that is set up for his or her special needs. We thought that if one had guests over one shouldn't have to feel that one's guests encroach on his or her personal space.

D. Cinelli. I think it's great. I think you've done a great job. I think you've done some very neat things that I really compliment you for. I guess pushing the envelope and being able to take the kind of notions of what's out there and being able to kind of layer it with the European communities and a lot of different things. For you to be able to talk about your culture, and say: "I'm not going to give up on being able to think that there are parts of my culture that can be adapted to people who graduated from the University of Michigan." I like the fact that you were able to say that this is my living room and this is a display or a place to be able to see people going by. The ability of a single-loaded mid-rise building versus a double loaded corridor, saying that a single loaded corridor maybe is more a function of a neighborhood. I really think that you've gone from macro to micro. You didn't solve all the problems, but what you looked at is saying that if I can solve this part on the site plan, and I can solve this part on the mid-rise, and I can solve this part on the duplexes. So, I really think you guys did a great job (Figure 8.7).

Michael. Thanks.

FIGURE 8.7. Jury Members Review the Project

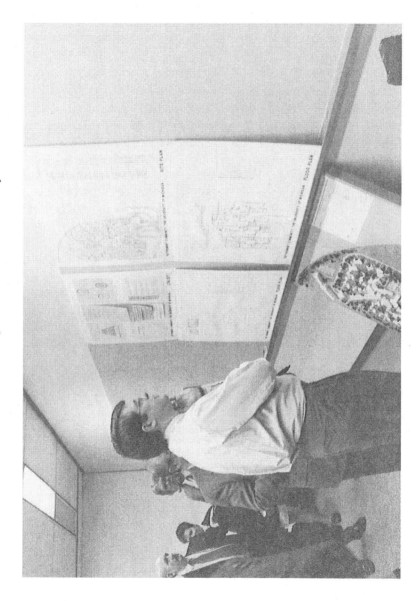

K. Brandle. I would agree with this in many, many ways. I like the centralization of your community. You have a real sense of community in that thing. I would have reinforced it with one other thing which I don't like in your scheme. And this is where you place this three or four-story apartment building. If you look at European schemes, you can see that this building could go right on top of the shops. Have you talked about that? Why don't you put that thing right here on top of that Main Street here? By doing this you have a community as much as you can get it. You can look down on the activities and you can increase by a considerable amount the land available for other uses. Also from an economic point of view it's important. Because I think as far as economics goes, I have real doubts with this shopping mall and all this for these few customers. I mean you have the support from the surrounding area, as we talked earlier, but you need more than that. I think you have to open it up so that people will really want to go there. You have to make sure that all the amenities here are viable economically. But I like the overall approach. I think it's very good.

G. Tipton. I'd like to reinforce both statements. I think that having the teamwork, perhaps, gave you more time to investigate in depth certain areas of your interest. I think it's a very good exploration of a lot of the issues, and very well resolved planning of a retirement community in the traditional sense. But you took it further, as Dan said. Because you've brought services into the community to make that a little more personal, yet you've brought services that reach to the larger community at large. I think that's really quite good. I do agree that the mid-rise should be located above Main Street. I had the feeling like there were two projects planned here that are kind of married in a forced marriage. The logical place would be right above. It seems like a logical connection because they're already living in a vertical way and that would give them direct access down into that space. Just as these folks are coming horizontally, they could go vertically. Otherwise I think all the aspects are solved. This is the kind of thing that I was hoping would be explored. I commend you for your effort to show how one unit could progress over a time as one's needs will change. Because this is the real essence of what we're struggling with here. How can you attract someone from a market point of view to move into a house that works well for them in good health and over time convert to something that's supportive of declining abilities. And also recognizing that they're going to have friends and guests who do not have those disabilities, and who have their needs. I think it's terrific in all these regards. Tying it back to the human needs and the psychological needs and reinforcing that diagrammatically is terrific. Well presented. You can understand how the thought process worked both in concept all the way through the presentation. I would like all the drawings to show a north arrow and a scale somewhere or another. Those are little pragmatic things that we worry about in the real world. One other real world thing; oftentime when you're tackling a problem and things just don't work, take some of the rules and just throw them out. You said that the lake or the ponds sit in this area and you put that over here. You just move some dirt around and you got a waiver from the Corps of Engineers and the Environmental Protection Agency, and they said: "That's okay. These guys have a great plan and it'll work." "What wet lands?" I do, I commend you. A lot of the really tough issues from the macro to the micro you tackled very well.

L. Knight. I commend you for being able to convert that garage space to something more useable for many people. The fact that you could make that into a caregiver's quarters, or student living or whatever is very nice. I think that particularly when someone lives alone and they need some more supportive services, they don't have a large enough apartment to accommodate that other person and that adaptation is a fantastic idea.

G. Tipton. There are lots of practical considerations from a cost point of view. The cost of care delivery is high. So saying, on the one hand, that a person's financial abilities are decreasing, yet their needs are increasing, having a live-in nurse brings a question of how much that costs. I mean the cost effectiveness of doing that is always going to be a question.

L. Knight. That's what the students are for. I think the opportunities for students, student nurses or social workers or activities directors, through internships in these communities would be fantastic.

G. Tipton. It addresses the whole question of what maybe a nursing home should become. It disappears, but it's integrated, which is very good. It is a reality of communities like this. The care needs to be delivered and ultimately that's why somebody does make the choice to move there. People just know that there will be some means by which care can be delivered. Maybe I'm never going to need it, but I want to make sure I know that in this environment, it can be there.

So, this is a way of getting rid of that awful nursing home environment and creating a new environment. You're exploring a new idea here which is quite good.

D. Cinelli. One micro point. As architects we're always so fixated about symmetry. And we only see things in plan. I'm wrestling with this right now for an Alzheimer's facility which has two separate wings. As the people here age in place, they still might be able to walk into the neighborhood. You might have some mild forms of dementia. The problem that you have is that if I have a mild form of dementia and I wander from the northeast side to the southwest side, it's completely the same. You flip-flop that corridor system and I'm going to try and go into a unit I think I live in, even though it's on the other side.

Michael. Interior finishes can help out.

D. Cinelli. It might even be shapes. It might be the configurations of those spaces. You have to be able to make those kinds of spaces totally different than the other side.

N. Levine. You've done something beautifully as far as a sense of scale is concerned. The next step that you would be taking from where you are at the present time is developing that even further. I'm looking at your pedestrian circulatory system, where you've built in what we call a semi-private type of space or semi-public type of space. That covered walkway wall can haunt you if you're not careful. In other words, it's covered to an extent, but legally you're going to be fighting every conceivable code in the world because of its potentially having a glass wall. Also the glass interfaces and how does it affect and impact upon its surrounding environment?

We recognize that you started with somebody that's independent and you've actually gone to an aging continuum. We're dealing with a factor that as we begin to age, we really build in a system of orientation to where we recognize we're at, what's going on. Hopefully as we begin to fail more and more, we begin to use a cueing process. We redundantly cue in on other factors that we will need. For example, if a person begins to wander or something like that we use the electronic system, that's a fabulous solution that you talked about. You've got to be careful as to how you do it. So that it doesn't become institutionalized to begin with as an end result. We went through a process just like this and as a matter of fact, I had a hell of an incident take place near the tail end of the project. We were in relocation which is a trauma to begin with, as far as an elderly person is concerned. We were walking through a court. As a matter of fact, I was walking with the dean of the college over here and ran into an individual. And I said: "Hello, how are you?" And she said: "I'm number 123." She forgot her name. So the dean said to me: "Well, Levine, you did a hell of a job over here. Not only does she not know who she is, but she became a number." So be very careful when you do the design process. System must become identifiable to the point. For example, the mailboxes are fabulous. That's clever. In fact, if you can identify that with something taken from their own home, it becomes an identifying cue to recognize where they're at. As you're changing space involved in a structure such as this. That's dynamic, that's fabulous. I commend you on doing a tremendous job of understanding human behavior as it integrates with the physical environment.

The site itself presented a beautiful view as far as taking those ponds out there and structuring the whole area. But what did you actually have in mind? Would you say that that's the interface with the community as a whole and is set forth as a major public space as an invitation for them to be able to come out and interface with the rest of the community? Your diagram again should be a 360 degree type of interface and it would illustrate what sort of a major impact you had as far as a major community area. It's a job, in my opinion, well done (Figure 8.8).

I do agree, the mid-rise is in a wrong location. If you study this site, it's in the highest part of the site. If anything, it wants to be brought down scale-wise to interface with the other buildings. And sitting within the context of the town center itself would give you something far more formidable and important. That's a hell of a long walk to the end of where you've got that last unit, all the way back into what we would call town center. Because you're structur-

FIGURE 8.8. The Team Reviews the Project

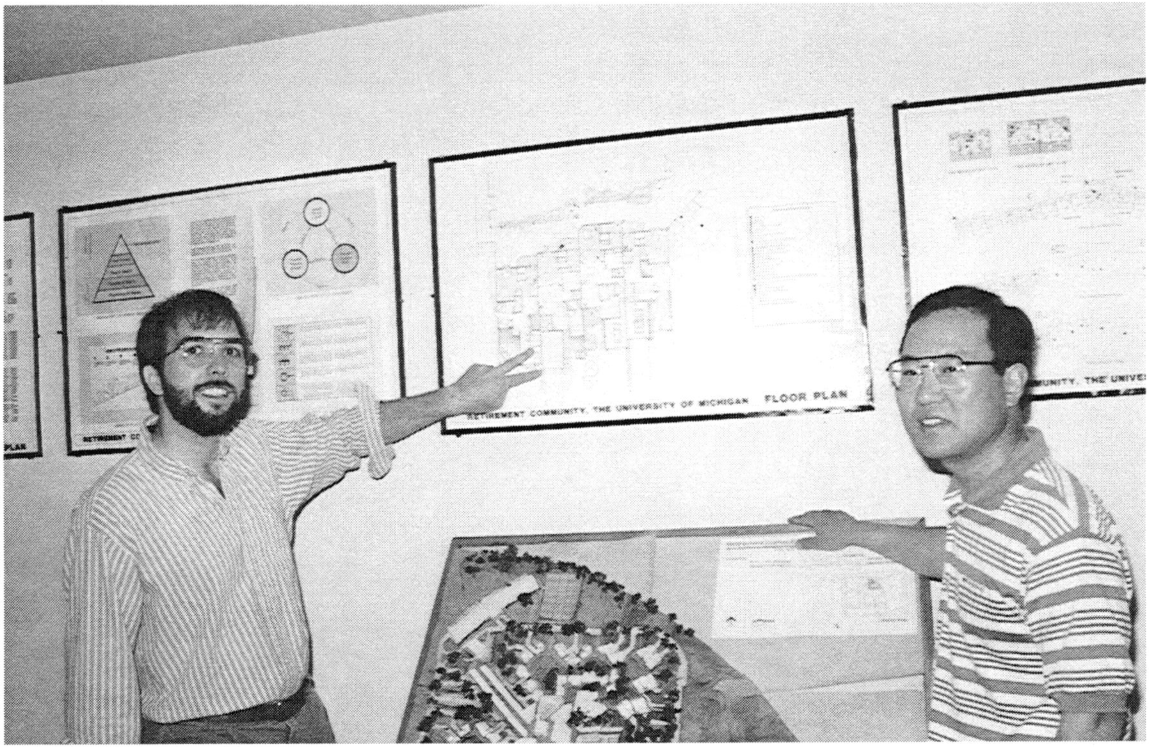

ing that building as a mid-rise, it's a congregate which stands on its own feet. Yet on the other hand you're saying: "I also want that to interface with the most structured environment, and the most intense area." Going vertically in that instance would give you a vertical circulation system that would have answered that question.

L. Pastalan. Jim Morgan has a rule of thumb for walking distance, no more than three minutes in the rain.

N. Levine. You're right.

G. Tipton. One minor point on the mailboxes. One of the reasons that mailboxes are in public areas is that it's a magnet to bring about socialization, to draw people out of their units to a common point earlier in the day rather than later in the day when the meals take place. I think that when the mail is delivered early and people go to retrieve their mail it promotes socialization. Because you walk along and meet people on their way and then you're there at a communal center and it's kind of a subtle prompting activity.

J. Hoadley. I think this project represents a recognition of the most intense health care services that you have to give. I like it in that it recognizes that when the health care and mobility of residents is at its lowest point, they still need to have 100% of life's quality available to them. But it shouldn't happen in their own place all the time. They definitely should be able to get it, and you recognize it by having covered walkways. You could actually phase this in by not building the public walkways and having to add the public walkways in. But the recognition that a person happens to be wheelchair bound completely, doesn't mean that they shouldn't go outside. You have to recognize that downtown becomes a place to go. One of the things in designing nursing homes, is that what you have is a captured resident. And a captured resident is entitled to every piece of life that you have when you're not a captured person in a building. They should be able to have different experiences just like you have in the real world. I think this captures that, it develops it to its most intense state. It would be interesting to see if you could, to really begin to study your next step. But I like the fact that you recognize that these people in their most, heaviest health needs really deserve a completed environment.

T. Hille. I have one statement to make. I agree with everything that's been said, in terms of the overall planning issue. The large scale and the small scale. The presentation and the site model are quite nice. But there is one question that I find really missing in this scheme. I'm interested in looking for images of what this place is actually like. Architecturally it bottoms out at some point and for a semester-long project I would expect that at some point you would have engaged that at an architectural level.

Michael. This is only a three credit hour class.

T. Hille. Well, I was afraid you were going to say something like that, and all I can say is there are ways that you can slice through the problem and at least get to it enough that you could imagine how the rest of it might be. This is typical of what might happen here, or this is typical of what it would look like as a transition from the street, from the house, and here's the materials and textures and light qualities and all of the things that architecturally I would find most exciting here. Most of the people here may think that other planning issues are more important. But, I guess I have a little bit of a question as you were going through your pyramid, where those issues fit in. Because things could be incredibly well planned and efficient and easy to use but that doesn't necessarily make it a wonderful apartment to live in. I would just like to see an inkling of that and I don't see it here.

D. Cinelli. You know what's interesting is that for a lot of architects who deal with the planning issues it is the main focus. To me the contextual elements of what things start to look like become so emotional. Also, my thoughts of what I thought it would look like, I've already envisioned in my head. To my mind I've already walked through this, and I've already envisioned what it looks like.

T. Hille. That is a good point. The reason I bring it up to these guys is because as a designer. As a designer I wouldn't leave that open ended.

G. Tipton. One interesting follow-up to that. In the first project that was presented the designer used an architectural element to connote residential, the arch. That appearance of the structure was very important in the overall cueing of what this place was all about.

I was curious as to what was in your thinking. You have a very decided contrast between the garage mass and very steep slopes of the cottages, contrasted with a very flat group of the Main Street.

What were your thoughts on this? I'm just curious as to what was behind these forms.

T. Hille. One last thing. The issue I'm bringing up is not an issue of style. It's an issue of what this place is in terms of habitation. These walls are massive, these walls are substantial. The roof plane hovers or is strongly grounded? These are important issues and I think this can easily be trivialized.

N. Levine. Your question really should ask: "Recognizing the team makeup and the two cultures, is it an adaptable philosophy on the basis of you both working on the project?" "Can you take it to your country and say: 1/10th of the philosophy is applicable to your life style? And if so, is it the same with you?" Because basically speaking, we're all human and we've all come into the world the same way and we leave the world the same way, and we live within the context of that as an environment wherever it may be. Because that's stylizing it. Whatever it may be, is really a facade. But in this instance, with the facade giving a feedback that it's applicable to the way you would live. Can you take this back to Korea and feel comfortable?

Kwang-Sun. Maybe.

Michael. Thank you very much.

Celebrating Life

Paul C. Ingman
Daniel Koester

Paul. First of all we'd like to thank Dr. Pastalan and Benny Schwarz for allowing us to be here with you and the rest of the class. We thank you and we thank our faculty members.

> (music)

> A friend of mine she cries at night
> and she calls me on the phone,
> Sees babies everywhere she goes
> and she wants one of her own.

> A friend of mine she cries at night and she calls me on the phone, Sees babies everywhere she goes and she wants one of her own.

> She's waited long enough she says
> and still he can't decide,
> Pretty soon she'll have to choose
> and it tears her up inside.

> She's scared, scared to run out of time

> I see my folks are gettin' on

[Haworth co-indexing entry note]: "Celebrating Life." Ingman, Paul C., and Daniel Koester. Co-published simultaneously in *Journal of Housing for the Elderly* (The Haworth Press, Inc.) Vol. 11, No. 1, 1994, pp. 145-168; and: *University-Linked Retirement Communities: Student Visions of Eldercare* (ed: Leon A. Pastalan, and Benyamin Schwarz) The Haworth Press, Inc., 1994, pp. 145-168. Multiple copies of this article/chapter may be purchased from The Haworth Document Delivery Center [1-800-3-HAWORTH; 9:00 a.m. - 5:00 p.m. (EST)].

and I watch their bodies change,
I know they see the same in me
and it makes us both feel strange.

No matter how you tell yourself
it's what we all go through,
Those lines are pretty hard to face
when they're staring back at you.

Scared to run out of time

When did the choices get so hard?
There's so much more at stake,
Life gets mighty precious
when there's less of it to waste.

Scared to run out of time[1]

Paul. Did you listen to those words? I guess we're trying to say that this is a pretty serious matter where people come here, not only to live but, possibly, to die. But on the other hand, we were trying to create a different image, an image that somehow inspires people to find dignity in their lives. We have tried to find humor and joy here. Spirit is what we're trying to create here. I think that traditionally we look at the artificial. We look at the economics, we look at the architectural details. And what we're saying here is that we want to look at nature first. I think this is the hierarchy that we evolved when we came into this world and is significant.

Dan. The song is inspiration. I think that's what we felt in the process. We had a lot of fun making it and going through this. What we wanted to emphasize was an Elders' Utopia. That's really the focus. How to make this fun, how to address people's lifestyles, wants, needs. What we've done schematically was to try and compact the research so that we can use that effectively throughout our design (Figures 9.1 and 9.2). We're thinking of nature as the primary inspiration for humanity.

One of the things that our people will want to accomplish in this

---

1. From *Nick of Time*, Bonnie Raitt. Published by Kokomo Music (ASCAP), 1989.

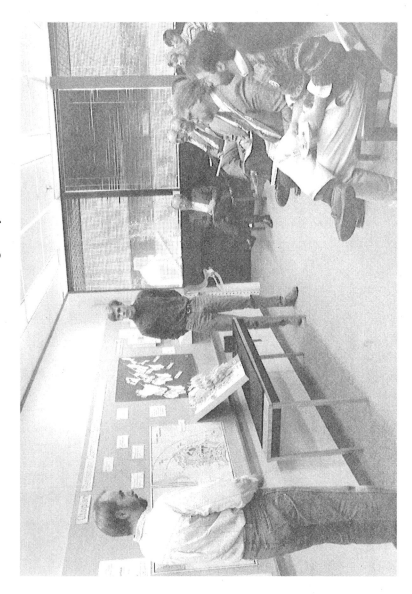

FIGURE 9.1. The Design Jury

FIGURE 9.2. Conceptual Plan

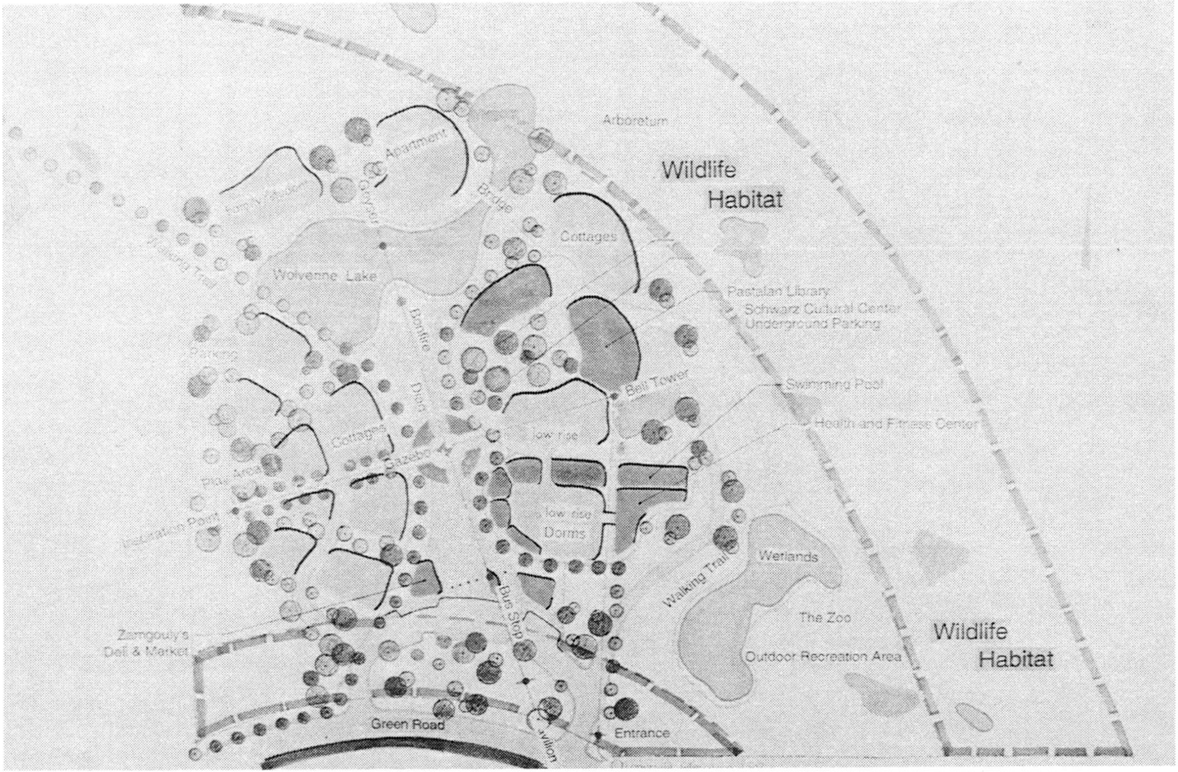

residency is to live longer by learning, through fitness, mental and physical health, and a sense of community. If you take the issue of aging in place I think that there's a lot of preconceptions about what we can do. What a nursing home is and what a nursing home can be. Part of this process of research is relearning for ourselves what's really possible. What are the true limitations? And what are the ones we impose on ourselves? I think that we've come up with some insights through that.

Paul. The word "connectedness." You're going to see that throughout our scheme. We started linking learning, community, fitness, the home. It's that kind of integration that we want to show. We want to get that kind of inspiration. We'd like to go quickly through the program. We invented this program. We talk about zoos with a llama corral. When we talk about the Schwarz graduate library or the Pastalan library, we're talking about education. We're talking about having fun. We're talking about an arboretum. We're talking about a diag. It's those kinds of fun things that we want to incorporate into our project. Things that make the community. That's the connectedness. Hopefully, we'll get the joy and happiness in this way.

We felt that nature is important. We have here a public park and we have a sugar bush park, down here where there's a soccer field and the kids can come. What we wanted to do is to create an envelope around this site which is basically already provided for us. There is a green belt outside on the freeway right of way. And we put in another green belt in here. What we wanted to do is to respect the high and the low lands, the wetlands. This demarcation line through here really represents elevation 950. This 950 line comes out just about where you'd want to provide some circulation or access into the site off Green Road. This is also 950. So it kind of provides almost a natural loop rising on both sides. If you've been on the site you notice that there are these nodes and they create this almost natural environment. We wanted to protect this. In the center of this we would hope to create this kind of Elders' Utopia (Figure 9.3).

So, preserving the wetlands, the natural areas, taking into consideration the circulation and then finding that flat area on the site. This would be the core. When I went to the site the first time, they

FIGURE 9.3. Site Analysis

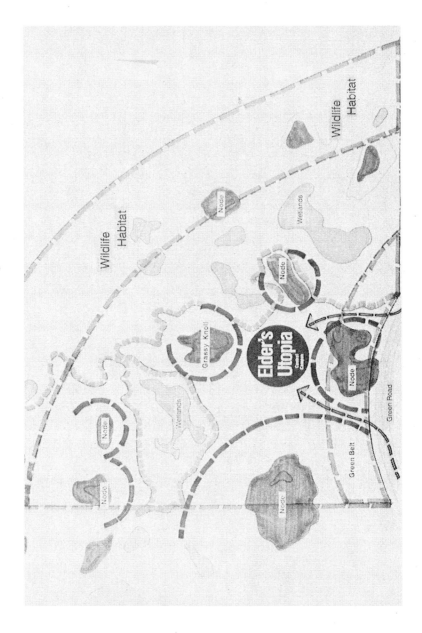

told me about all the traffic noise there. I got out of the car, and it was January, snowy, and I couldn't hear the noise. The reason I couldn't hear was due to the birds. The birds were so noisy. And all over the snow were all these tracks. I don't know what they were, but there were tracks there. So we want to protect that. We think that's an attribute of the site, the wildlife that's already there. We want to make that part of this joy, excitement and this image that the elders should have when they come here.

Dan. The other thing is bringing it back to the campus of the University of Michigan. I think that's reflected in the program. We can move on to how we developed the site schematically. The main emphasis was a pedestrian core than ran straight through the site paved with cobblestone. We are calling that a Diag area. To the left of that is off-campus housing which are one bedroom units that are bunkered into that hill that gradually slopes up. To the right of the Diag is our central campus, which is our model.

One of the aspects that's been mentioned today that we also hoped would happen is that students would become part of this community. Maybe it's health professionals working in nursing or social workers who would find a part-time job or some benefit in living here as opposed to another part of campus. This part would be families also. Less for undergraduate students, and more for graduate students with families.

Paul. There's a bus stop down on Green Road. We'd like to place that bus stop here and this becomes a hub for this community. We'd like people from the neighborhood to come here, the children to go to the market to buy their bubble gum or whatever when they go to the park. The pedestrian access off of Green Street can lead you into this public park. People from the public park back around under the Diag can go around Wolverine Lake across and maybe back into this arboretum where the wildlife is. I think there's real potential for ex-faculty members who might be botanists or biologists to participate and enhance the wildlife in this area. It's that kind of integration with nature, with the community. I see these people having an opportunity to baby-sit for these people in this area or that kind of mix.

Dan. As many levels as possible to extend the University to this site and the people here back to the University.

Paul. And again, that's the connectedness we're speaking about. Trying to tie it in to every level, the community, the natural environment.

Dan. We find that on what we've called the graduate library and the cultural center. These areas where a person who lives here, who is an alumni who has come back to the University, can spend potentially reorienting back to what campus life is like. How you get to classes, how you CRISP, how the bus system works.

I was talking with a woman who was 75 years old and audited classes in auditoriums at the University. And a rush of undergraduate students would come in and she would almost be knocked over. She ended up dropping the course. So I think there are potentials to bring some of that up here and also maybe ways of dealing with those kinds of frustrations of going back into the University setting.

We're at 950 which is the Diag level and we see the front part of this as administration and retail shops and a coffee shop. Things that would take advantage of that view up the knoll to the other side. There's a road that's coming in the site that ends up at 940 level. This is where the underground parking will be, at 940 and above that at 950 with a circular drive to connect the two. The level above that, 960, this grassy knoll that's coming up across here, puts us at the cultural center. We see a swimming pool actually at the 950 level that has a glass or open space above. This is the health fitness center. This is a place where we have trainers. If you have an injury or you're rehabilitating there's facilities to help you as well as a swimming pool and regular gym equipment.

We have on this bank what we're calling the Wolverine Inn which looks out over Wolverine Lake and that could have a couple of purposes. It allows people to come in. Maybe if you were just thinking about, do I want to move to retirement in a sense, or what's that going to be like? My vision is that if a person stays in this for a day and comes up to the fourth floor dining facility and sees the piano bar and the four-star dining, they're going to get a positive feeling about what this community is like and what the potentials are.

Paul. As well as visitors.

Dan. Who might be coming for Saturday Football. We picture this as booked a year in advance. And on Saturday morning they go up and watch the cars pile on U.S. 23 coming into town.

Paul. When you look at this green, there aren't any roofs. If you looked at this project from the air, you would see no roofs because what we hope to have here is roof gardens and roof terraces where people can come out of their back door onto these roof terraces (Figure 9.4).

Now this model has been expanded so you can see inside of it. But if compressed the intent would be that somehow we could walk up onto these, so we're going to challenge the elderly to do that.

Dan. There are interior elevators at two locations on the site. There's one here, here and here. And then exterior stairways linking the roof gardens. It's not a concept that we've resolved, but potentially in your backyard you have a back door with a fenced off garden area with a path. There may be paths that develop through here so that you could walk in the front and get to the back of the building just on roof gardens.

Here are the two bedroom units which are primarily what we have on campus (Figure 9.5). Off campus would be the one-bedroom cottages.

Paul. We tried to standardize the units. But we feel that there is a need to make those with some kind of individual orientation. Not to create a corridor where they all back up with some tunnel effect with no windows. We felt that we need to fenestrate not only the corridor, but also the outside. And so what we were trying to create in this model is that somehow we can look into the public corridor space with glass and look through. We're not going to get hung up on how to make that glass or how that detail would work. I think as architects we can come up with something or maybe modify something. But the intent, the image that we're trying to create is that we can look through. It can create a problem if we have a public corridor in a private space, how do we handle that. So we don't really have a solution here. I know that. But these are the kinds of things that we would want to happen here.

We created almost a shared semi-public space. If you come up and look at the model, we've created what we call a water wall. So that when someone is in the public corridor and goes through that space, they're going to see the natural light coming through that,

FIGURE 9.4. Conceptual Model of Housing Cluster

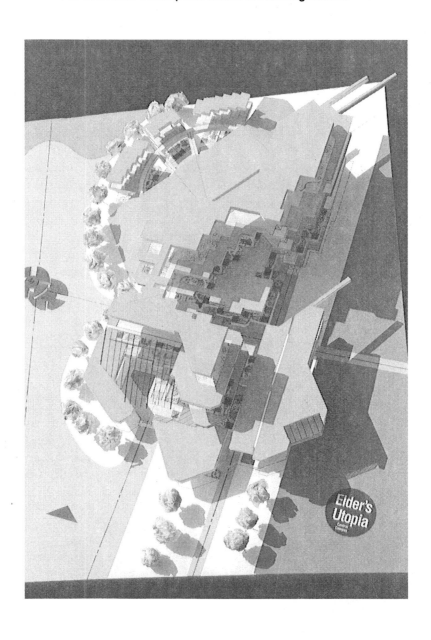

FIGURE 9.5. A Floor Plan for Two Bedroom Condo

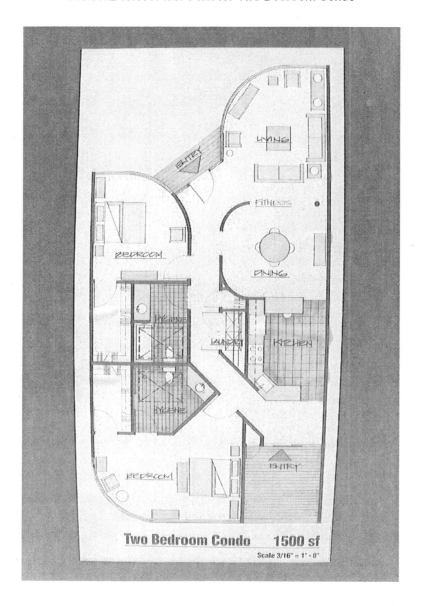

reflecting off the water. They can hear the noise, and they can see the movement of the water and then the trees hopefully grow over this kind of space. It's kind of an experiential happening for them, not only in the public way, but in the semi-public space (Figure 9.6).

Dan. Another element that we've tried to consider throughout this, is the idea of fitness. It's part of thinking of how we approach this type of community. Do we look at it in terms of nursing care or do we look at it in terms of health and fitness and working out and swimming. So we've included here in both of these units an area for fitness. It's in a public area.

Fitness isn't something you tuck in and you slide your rowing machine out from under your bed once a month and do a few reps. It's something that's a part of your lifestyle. Something that you do in between cooking meals, something you can interact with while watching TV.

This is a related project that I'm doing with Ron Sekulski and it's looking at one issue, rising from a chair. Elderly people report having problems getting up out of a chair. This is a device that we can create that they can use. This looks like it's appropriate for their home, like a piece of furniture, that they interact with and strengthen the muscles that you would use to rise from a chair. This sketch model. But the idea is that you can sit on this. There's a spring and a piston in there, and it will lower you down. It's giving you weight, it's supporting you while you sit. It would be adjustable if you are heavier or lighter. This is one concept attached to a pole. This is more traditional exercise prescribed, a low tech thing, you can do with the chair. Things with stepping. If this were done in conjunction with a pole that you could hold in front of you, it could have created a more stable situation. It's a concept that we create. A new space in the residence that's dedicated to health and fitness.

Paul. We have a little tape we'd like you to listen to. That is our feeling of what it should be like if you lived here.

(music)

By the shores of old Lake Michigan
where the hawk winds blow so cold,

FIGURE 9.6. Conceptual Model of Apartment Cluster

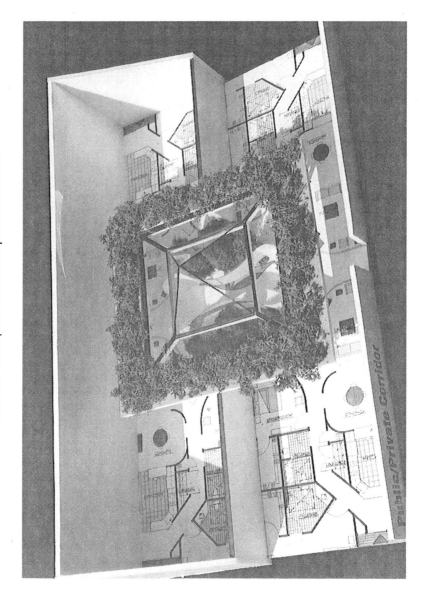

An old Cub fan lay dying
in his midnight hour of the toll.

On his bed his friends had all gathered
they knew his time was short,
And on his head they put this bright blue cap
from his all-time favorite sport.

He told them, It's late, its getting dark here
and I know it's time to go,
but before I leave the line-up
there's one thing I'd like to know.

Do they still play the Blues in Chicago
when Baseball season rolls around?
When the snow melts away, do the Cubbies
still play in their ivy covered burial grounds?
When I was a boy they were my pride and joy
but now they only bring fatigue,
To the home of the free, the land on the brave,
and the doormat of the National League.

He told his friends, You know the law of averages
says anything will happen that can,
But the last time the Cubs won a National League
         Pennant
was the year we dropped the bomb on Japan.

The Cubs made me a criminal, they put me down
         a wayward path,
they stole my youth from me, that's the truth.
I'd forsake my teachers to sit in the bleachers
         in flagrant truancy.

And one thing lead to another and soon I discovered
         alcohol,
gambling, dope, football, hockey, lacrosse;
But what do you expect when you raise up a young
         boy's hopes

and then crush them like so many paper beer cups.
Year after year after year. . . .
Till those hopes are just so much popcorn
    for the pigeons
beneath the L-tracks to eat.

He said, You know, I'll never see Wrigley field
    anymore
before my eternal rest,
So if you have your pencil and scorecards ready
I'll read you my last request:

Give me a double header funeral in Wrigley field
    on some sunny weekend day, no lights,
Have the organ play the National Anthem and a little
Nah, Nah, Nah, Nah, Hey, Hey, Hey, Goodbye

Make six bullpen pitchers carry my coffin
and six groundskeepers clear my path,
Have the umpires bark me out at every base
in all their holy wrath.

It's a beautiful day for a funeral,
hey Ernie, let's play too,
Somebody get Jack Brickhouse to come back
to conduct just one more interview.

Have the Cubbies run right out onto the field
have Keith Moreland drop a routine fly,
Give everybody two bags of peanuts and a frosty malt
and I'll be ready to die.

Build a big fire at home base out of your
Louisville sluggers and toss my ashes in,
Let my ashes blow in a beautiful snow
from the 30 mile per hour southwest winds.

And when my last remains fly over the left field wall
we'll bid the bleacher bums adieu,

And I will come to my final resting place
out on Waitland Avenue.

The dying man's friends told him to cut it out
they said stop it, that's an awful shame,
He whispered Don't cry, we'll meet by and by
near the heavenly Hall of Fame.

He said, I've got season tickets to see the angels now
so it's just what I'm going to do,
And he said, But you the living are stuck here
        with the Cubs
so it's me that feels sorry for you.

Play that lonesome losers tune,
that's the one I like to hear,
close his eyes and slipped away,
It was the dying Cub's fan's last request;
and here it is,

Do they still play the Blues in Chicago
when baseball season rolls around?
When the snow melts away, do the Cubbies
still play in their ivy covered burial grounds?
When I was a boy they were my pride and joy
but now they only bring fatigue,
To the home of the free, the land on the brave,
and the doormat of the National League.[2]

G. Tipton. One thing that Dan (Cinelli) and I immediately
grasped the second we walked in the door is the one thing we
haven't talked about at all today, which is a major part of this
industry. And this is marketing. Everybody talked about it this
morning, why would someone be inclined to become involved in
this. Well, you've seized upon this opportunity to market your
concept to us. And a lot of this creating the visual and the sound
environment, putting us on your team, quotes from the members of

2. *A Dying Cub Fans Last Request* by Steven Goodman. Red Pajama Re-
cords, 1983.

the jury, it is all marketing. It is a very big part of what makes these communities succeed or fail.

You really made a point of the connectedness by connecting this to the site. The fact that you have integrated the buildings with nature (Figure 9.7). The fact that you planned the site with the lakes that are there, you've accepted it. The previous scheme did a very good job of exploring a lot of the issues of doing retirement communities. But effectively they ignored the reality of that site. You very much knitted it with the site, which I think is quite successful. I also commend you on trying to explore a variation on more traditional housing types that you expect to see in this arena.

There are a lot more intricate parts of this that we talked about earlier today that I'm kind of curious about. For instance, the delivery of care to the units. We talked about aging in place. I'm sure this would be thrilling for a person to live and that you would die with the same joy for life that our Cub's fan did in the presentation, but can you tell me how someone would age in place here and how you would provide services to them over the continuum of their life?

Dan. I can start. I would first note that the units are totally wheelchair accessible and you've heard already about the cabinets that raise and lower. But, I want to address your marketing issue first. I feel the positive side of marketing is education and I think what we tried to do was to say that there is a preconceived notion of what a retirement community is. And there are elements here of life-long learning, fitness, nature that maybe will create a different type of model. It's a step of getting away from preconceptions to something else. In the same way, we created a unit that is totally wheelchair accessible. Everything here is wheelchair accessible.

We visited a retirement community that had a floor that had two accessible rooms. Everything else was catch as catch can. If you look at other models, Scandinavia for example, you find nurses riding bikes to people's units. There are indoor corridors that allow for bicycle transportation. So I think that there are delivery models that are out there that will change our perspective of pulling a person out of their room and putting them in nursing. Having a floor that is centered around nursing stations as opposed to living units is not our idea of retirement community. We talked about mobility for the elderly population. How many elderly people really are pre-

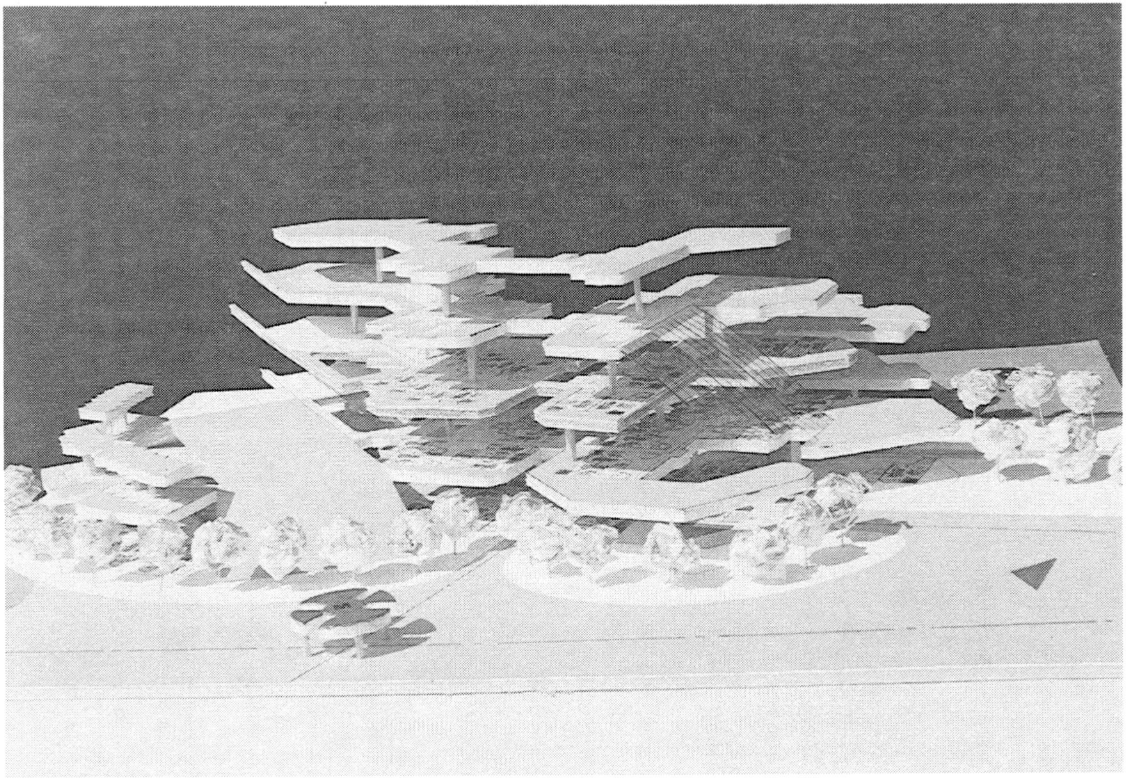

FIGURE 9.7. Side View of the Conceptual Model of the Housing Cluster

scribed power wheelchairs? Not many, because Medicare won't pay for it. So there are issues that society needs to address. Mobility could be much more diverse. There could be a bed you could drive around; if someone would just invent it, someone else would pay for it. I think there's the potential for new things.

N. Levine. I really like the approach in your project. I recognize that it's marketing. But the way to build a facility is to look at the positive aspects of life in order to stress those. I really believe that in retirement facilities we should have a word like Elder's Utopia. It should have all these great things. That's what they should be. That's how we should be. This is a place for people to live.

The idea is to stress the positive part of life and the excitement of living and capturing the emotions. This is really, this is doing this. I like that. It's looking at it from a wide point of view, not a care point of view. I think you can apply the care to that kind of environment. But I find this very exiting, I like this. It is very refreshing. We could design some nursing homes with this input or similar to this. I think it's really something. If you want to attract somebody to live in a place, this is how you approach the design as well as the marketing. You cannot market it if you didn't do this to the design. It will fail. So I think, we can go after the little parts and things like that, but I think the concept is very, very nice. As professionals we need to look at things like this and go away saying, "That's right." If you forget that you lose the emotion of your facility, you lose the emotion of life. And retirement facilities are places where people live and this is lifestyle.

K. Brandle. I would agree with all that was said. I would like to have, however, a little bit of better connection between the units, which are fine and very interesting. I would like to know how the building really works. Not the total design. But there is a little bit of gap here. I feel I don't know how these things really work. How these non-corridors, as you describe them, how they work. In the model this is kind of nice that everybody can have a waterfall. Whether you can afford it is a different story. But I really don't know how that works. And this is very crucial. I mean I see that you have a kind of a little mountain of a building, which is fine. But I would like to see a little bit more how these things work vertically.

Another thing is from a viability point of view. How many units do you have in that?

Paul. Just let me preface that by saying that we felt that you could get up to a certain point, there has to be some economic viability here or this doesn't fly.

K. Brandle. You have a huge piece of land and a very small amount of units.

Paul. Right. And in consideration of your last statement, we feel the people should be participants in this design process. So in the main campus area right now we have 75 units, and we think we could handle 500 in these outside areas. Maybe we could handle more than that. It depends on the design. We think that the residents should be participants. All we showed, basically, was the site schematic. And we showed these, clusters. In the main campus we have what we call the dorms. Those are all two bedroom units. And we're trying to get the 80-20 mix. That's what our thinking was.

G. Tipton. Don't misconstrue my comments as being negative. I applaud the creative thinking and the way you developed a program and knitted that with the diagrammatic approach to site planning and knitted that with the natural features of the site. And then almost jumped from that very broad-based thinking to a very detailed thing. There's something in between that I think we're struggling to understand a little bit better. There's all sorts of details in communities like this that you worry about that probably should be at least commented on. So that with wonderful ideas you don't wind up somehow losing sight of a couple of things the elderly might quite literally trip over. Like, for instance, a cobblestone major pedestrian way, if there weren't an alternative way of getting to a place. They might say, "Gee, this is great to look at, but I can't walk any distance without falling"; or "I love this south facing area that's glazed here, but with the glare that's associated with it I really don't want to walk out into the corridor, because of the contrast between the light there and here." All those kinds of issues that are somewhere between this broad-based concept and the details of that plan.

Paul. We'd like to say that you're right and that was one of the frustrations. This thing is so big. We didn't have the time to make that leap so you get a sense of what we're trying to do at the end. It was difficult for me to get to that point without going through those things.

N. Levine. I think what you have really accomplished is that you looked at something starting right off with a problematic site and you excited yourself to the extent of saying: "I'm dealing with a specific phase of a program and I really design something that would interface with that." What you've done is grasp the inherent qualities of the ecology of the site itself. You've picked the worst part of the site and said: "Let me see if I can do this and handle this both vertically as well as horizontally, as far as a movement of a human being." What you've actually accomplished is that excitement that you've built up within the program of understanding what you're dealing with. The excitement of what you've started with is the keynote facility which offers all of the amenities that can forthwith and all of the various clusters in other parts of that community that you're playing with. You're building upon the key building to state, "I think there's something here that I haven't seen before. I would like to live here." Now the development of the plan that you're dealing within the infrastructure of the multi-story structure is that you have pushed that to the extremities. I can move in at any given age but I've also taken into consideration that I have mobility to the extent where I may possibly end up in the context of a wheelchair. So you've structured that facility to where you've taken your vertical orientation and kept everything close knit, and you're utilizing your vertical transportation system to take people down to your central support area. That's beautiful.

The levels of where you're interfacing the site ecology with the levels of education, where you can almost have a built-in horticultural therapy program–there you've got something that's exciting; that's ongoing all the time within the infrastructure and out to the outer extremities of the building. And the building itself, leveling off with the contours of the land. You've taken the other nodes of activity to expand upon the potential of its economics. Just how you can push it with an alternative type of units, whether it be clusters of housing that interface with this type of thought process or another, is something else. What you are telling me is that there's innovativeness, there's cleverness, there's understanding of program. There's an understanding of site ecology and expressing what is futurism. We may be seeing facilities which you've taken a real charge at and developed. You've taken a problematic site and really done a heck of a number. You understand that site beautifully. The general contours of that site. Where you enter. You've allowed for major entry, reception type of area. You've given them a mode of pedestrian movement as well as vehicular. You've captured the quality site with various lakes. You've given them titles of dignity. And what you did you did right from the beginning. You set forth a theme of who your occupants may become. You have structured the program to the cultured environment emanating from the University saying, "I've got something that may even excite you, as you grow older, to want to live at something very innovative and very unique." I think you did a very commendable job.

G. Tipton. You could also attract younger people just on the basis of its uniqueness and exciting switch, you know, in and of itself marketing. I don't mean to trivialize that at all.

Paul. I think that's an important point. We were hoping to have the kids that would interface with some elderly persons who would then invite them to their homes. You'd get that mix going. Because there really are attractions here. The bowling alley, or the chip and putt golf course . . .

D. Cinelli. I'd like to say something. I feel like I've been over-marketed in the presentation. I think that as you go out and you practice, you do have to make a presentation to a client. You have to be careful that you don't put them down or you don't over-market them. Because what happens is that, I feel like you're pulling something over on me and I start looking at some of the cuteness of this project and I miss some of the most important points that you're trying to get across. I think you've got to really be careful.

You pointed to this word called connectedness. Graphically this project is not connected and there is a skip over and some skips that almost become reverse apparent to me. I mean, that isolated points of what I'm seeing here graphically are very nice. But, when I start to try to put these together there is no correlation of green on the reverse board. There is no correlation of green on the two-bedroom condos. There is no section for me to understand where the corridor is. So you've given me snapshots but there's no common thread. I think it's a great project and you kind of combine here deconstruction in a way. I think that, if you just look at that piece in isolation and say, this is an experiment and this is how this went, I think it works. But I think you've got to be really careful because one could really feel hoaxed.

Paul. I was concerned about that. You're absolutely right. I was concerned that we were going to hammer you with those. So, I respect your comments very much. I'm concerned about the comment about the M. I'm hoping that the Michigan Symphony would play there. I see glass and this gazebo and people would be drawn to the outside of this. It may be filled with music in the air and those kinds of things. And when the geyser on July 4th you can see the lights. I mean, this could be a real hub of the community. But you're right, these are snapshots. There should have been better visual coordination between these elements.

K. Brandle. This drawing is really very hard to read. And remember that eventually you have to sell the project not to architects. You have to sell it to a client who doesn't have that sophistication of connecting as we do, hopefully, to some extent. When I see a drawing like this I have a hard time at the moment to see what connectedness does as a plan. It's very hard to make the step from here to here. A client may not be able to make that kind of link between these various things.

Paul. I would never do this to a client. I'm hoping you can see that we're trying to get the image across and we're not trying to deal with architectural details which I could draw for you.

G. Tipton. The jury experience is very, very helpful in preparation for a presentation to a client, because it's really your best preparation for presenting the entire story of how you developed the design and so on. Dan's point is well taken.

N. Levine. There's good conceptual thinking here.

G. Tipton. You're exploring new directions and you've presented in a different way. I find that encouraging but Dan's point is very well taken.

L. Knight. I was just going to comment that when you were doing the presentation I felt that this would be a fun place to go. I mean, I could live here easily. And I was thinking about a lot of different aspects of this concept that would appeal to me at this stage of my life. This is the first time I've ever really thought about a community in that way, that it would be fun. I thought it would be a kind of whimsy and have all the elements that I think are important for the quality of my life.

Dan. To quote Lee, in concept it's a land-based cruise ship.

K. Brandle. I think what it achieves, and that is maybe why we talk, is that it's not really a community for the elderly necessarily. You said this a few times, and this is very positive. Very positive, because while it is basically planned for older people, it has a lot of interesting aspects to it, which could draw people around 50 or so.

D. Cinelli. What's interesting about this concept is that if you think about a utopian society there are no age barriers. There is also no stylistic type of attitude to the building. It kind of makes one shed any stylistic notions about what home is about. Whether or not one came from a Victorian ranch-house or a colonial ranch-house. It makes you want to take off the style coat and say: "Here I am. I'm about all these things that you want to put me through. I'm ready for that. I'm ready to just kind of walk into the waters of this project and shed everything I've got because I've lived in a university town." I think this is the final knock on the head saying, "don't think about housing as something that is a vernacular of the home you've been living in all your life." This makes a nice translation into that thinking.

H. Naimark. One additional dimension to add, and this is a hope, we don't feel like it's a dead end. You expressed a unique feeling here. Learning and fitness and there's something very upbeat about it. If there is anything that people feel in retirement communities it is that there is no hope, there's no more left in life. And I think this place is different.

AFTERWORD

Emergent Themes

Leon A. Pastalan
Benyamin Schwarz

Several themes evolved during the design and the review process of this volume. The concept of *community* is, perhaps, a predominant one. The usage of the term *community* is associated with a certain ambiguity because of its several meanings. In his classic review of 94 definitions of community found in the literature, Hillery (1955) noted that the three most commonly mentioned elements are: (1) social interaction; (2) common ties in the sense of shared values; and (3) a geographical area. Analysis of a community from a designer's perspective leads to the realization that it consists of dwellings and shops, of places for work and education, meeting and recreation. It harmonizes systems of communication and other human needs.

University-Linked Retirement Communities was expected to focus on the architectural aspect of its structures as well as on its

[Haworth co-indexing entry note]: "Emergent Themes." Pastalan, Leon A., and Benyamin Schwarz. Co-published simultaneously in *Journal of Housing for the Elderly* (The Haworth Press, Inc.) Vol. 11, No. 1, 1994, pp. 169-178; and: *University-Linked Retirement Communities: Student Visions of Eldercare* (ed: Leon A. Pastalan, and Benyamin Schwarz) The Haworth Press, Inc., 1994, pp. 169-178. Multiple copies of this article/chapter may be purchased from The Haworth Document Delivery Center [1-800-3-HAWORTH; 9:00 a.m. - 5:00 p.m. (EST)].

169

policies and programs. The students attempted to emphasize the relationship between design and residents' satisfaction. Their projects addressed the identity of the community, its physical boundaries, the social networks, the concentrated use of area facilities, and the special emotional and symbolic connotations for its future inhabitants. In their own way, the students tried to blend concepts of Howard's *Garden City* with constructs from the small town America. Piazzas, squares, and street patterns played a significant role in the pedestrian environment that was postulated in each of the projects. Small retail shops, personal businesses, and services such as banks, post offices, health care offices, etc., were incorporated into the site plans. Combinations of employment and residential uses with recreational and educational facilities were blended into the utopian retirement community as the students attempted to capture the qualities of a small town.

AGE-SEGREGATED VERSUS AGE-INTEGRATED COMMUNITY

The second theme that evolved during the design process was the issue of age-segregated versus age-integrated and diversified community. Typically, retirement communities are structured as age-segregated settings which make them by definition not ordinary homes. Contrary to the *Disengagement* theory which dominated the sociology of aging in the past, there has been growing awareness among researchers that residential development for older people cannot be viewed or experienced as typical, for age-segregation itself sets such places apart from the norm. Nevertheless, for some elderly it may be a very satisfying situation as evidenced by a number of studies. People tend to want to have some commonality in interests and capabilities or level or styles of living. There are also older people who choose to live in retirement communities simply because they enjoy living and socializing with others their age and participating in organized leisure and recreational activities. Golant (1992) summarized the four major reasons for attraction to continuing care retirement communities as they appear in the literature:

- A feeling of personal security in the event that help is needed on an emergency basis.
- The prospects of living independently in an attractive setting in secure, private living quarters requiring minimum upkeep.
- The contractual guarantee that health services and personal and nursing home care will be available when needed and that there is financial protection against the catastrophic costs of long-term care.
- A desire not to be a burden on one's children or friends, or expressed more positively, the appeal to managing and being in control of one's own life. (p. 264)

Our democratic instincts reject age-segregated communities which may disclose patterns of ageism, or as one of the students called it, "the internal walls that we build in our society." Aging in the American society is perceived often as a problem. Aging is seen as a nuisance, or a burden that has to be taken care of. American society glorifies youth and independence and has fears of weakness, dependency, and disease. These attitudes are reflected in several forms of segregation such as: social policies toward elderly people, allocation of resources, planning of services and other forms of what our society regards as solutions to the "problem" of aging.

The idea of a university-linked retirement community reflects the wish to create an intergenerational mix. It appears beneficial to the young as well as to the old, for it helps young people overcome their fears of growing old, it helps them to understand the life-cycle and to understand that older persons are, first, persons, and only second, they happen to be old.

Most of the students involved in this book tried to address these issues by opening their site-plans to the surrounding community. They wanted to avoid the isolation by incorporating restaurants open to the public and child care facilities to attract younger age groups. Moreover, all the projects included educational facilities for mixed age students. Their purpose was to introduce education for *all* students regarding the biological, social, and psychological changes of the lifecycle; the social problems of age-status and age-group expectations. However, at the same time, the projects recognized the rights of some old and some young to prefer same-age peer groups by creating different options for both old and young.

AGING IN PLACE

Another theme was *aging in place.* That is the concept of remaining within the same residential setting throughout various stages of aging without the need to relocate to other facilities even as the residents may experience age-related cognitive and physical changes. Separation of different levels of shelter and care is a common practice in the design and management of CCRCs. Residents of retirement communities are expected to move from one part of the CCRC to another as their needs for services and consequent living arrangements change. During her or his tenure a resident can conceivably occupy a rental apartment in the independent accommodations of a congregate housing facility, a room for the semi-dependent in an assisted living center, and a double occupied room in a skilled nursing home.

Site plans of CCRCs reflect the segmentation of shelter and care. Nursing facilities are frequently hidden in the rear of the property, far away from the main entrance. The common justifications are: More able residents prefer not to mingle with the less competent because they may associate physical proximity to frail aged as personal closeness to death and dying; independent elderly do not want to be aligned with an environment which projects an image of a hospital. People fear becoming institutionalized. The basic anxiety for many older people about long-term care is the fear of being forced to move to a nursing home when they become too frail to manage themselves and to reside permanently in a custodial facility that is not home. Nursing homes are often seen as society's predominant solution for dealing with those aged and disabled among us who are unfortunate enough to outlive their social and economic usefulness. However, several CCRC residents may need long-term care services as they age and the nature of long-term care accommodations in the retirement community is critical. Residents must agree to the rules of the CCRC which frequently include restrictions regarding the occupancy and use of apartments or rooms as well as the medical and disability situation. Based upon these restrictions they are expected to relocate to more supportive accommodations within the CCRC. And these are not normal residences, nor are they desirable ones.

Building on these notions the students' projects displayed different solutions to the continuum of care. Most of them have been attracted to some form of *aging in place*. Several of them liked the Scandinavian models of eldercare where in recent years the *nursing home* concept was replaced by *home nursing*. The philosophical basis for this concept is the maximization of functional independence for all the residents by providing long-term health-care guarantees through a pooled-risk arrangement to the residents. Yet unlike the common CCRC, this solution promises the occupants can maintain their own housing arrangements on the site with services that allow them to continue to live independently as long as it is possible or practical. The students envisioned that residents of their projects had a contract that was expected to provide for a comprehensive range of services under the management of the retirement community. These services were guaranteed for as long as the contract remained in effect or for the lifetime of the residents. Design solutions that followed this form of continuum of care grappled with several problems which included but were not restricted to: How to deliver and to coordinate adequate service for residents who are geographically dispersed? How to monitor residents' health situation and deliver services when they are needed? How to strike a balance between residents' needs and cost-effectiveness? What are the best physical expressions of this service delivery system?

ENVIRONMENT-BEHAVIOR DESIGN: A MEETING PLACE FOR DISCIPLINES

A design course such as the one described in this book has its own limitations. The major one is *time*. In their effort to explore more deeply the alternatives for their elders' utopia a few of the students ran out of time and could not develop architectural elevations and sections which would have helped them to better explore the nature of the places they designed. Some members of the jury referred to these deficiencies. Others thought that these were minor issues and felt that as professionals in this field they have the capability to envision the designed places even without further details. Another "shortcoming" of this course was embedded in its structure. Most design studios and design juries imply that the students' primary responsibility is to the profession of architecture. However, this studio was based on the environment-behavior paradigm. Consequently, the emphasis of the educational process shifted toward the imaginary occupants, or the users. This move frequently results in the structure of the course, in the selection of the required readings, in the nature of the design jury, and in the selection of the jurors.

The paradigm of environment-behavior design has transfused architectural studies for more than 30 years now. Both the need for theoretical understanding of the relationship between people and their surroundings and immediate, pragmatic concern over mismatch between people, institutions, communities and designed environments have provided impetus for this paradigm. This model, which was based on the conflation of social sciences and architecture, focused on human beings, who occupied buildings and communities, the users. A number of architects and social scientists have anticipated that by incorporating social-behavioral sciences into the architectural design process, the resulting buildings would function better for users and occupants. That's maybe a romantic notion but we still hold to it.

The sub-field of environment and aging developed from the same awareness of the two-way character of the transaction between the person and the environment. Still, from its early stages, it dealt with the reality that the elderly are, statistically speaking, more vulnerable to environmental pressures than the young and therefore, the impact of deficits in the environment on their behavior is greater (Lawton & Simon, 1968). There is no doubt that this focus on the functional aspects of person-environment relations in late life has generated important insights. Nevertheless, the functional orientation ignored meaningful facets of elderly peoples' lives. As Lawton (1987) noted:

> The docility and proactivity conceptions underline what I see as a basic dialectic in conceptualizing services for the elderly: support versus autonomy. Decline and deprivation demand

support, but the human spirit demands autonomy. The view that either aspect of this duality tells the whole story is sheer fantasy. Proactive environments, such as institutions, were not constructed to crush human spirit but to attempt to adjust the average press level of vulnerable people to one consistent with their competence. Our errors have come in assuming that all forms of press are negative and that autonomy ends once competence is low enough to require a specialized environment. (p. 37-38)

The goal of the architects in the field of environment and aging has been to find approaches to environmental design that take into account the fact that aging, particularly extreme old age, does bring physical and sensory limitations that alter one's ability to negotiate the environment. For this reason architects have used experts in psychology and sociology of aging to translate these special needs into space lists and design programs. The problem with these programming lists is that too often they are merely functional-oriented, and their outcomes, with few exceptions, are environments that afford no links with one's personal or cultural past. Most residential care facilities for the elderly, particularly those which are closer to the more institutional end of the scale, are environments in which individuals have very limited opportunities to assert personal meaning. Thus the real challenge for designers is to be able to recognize environmental attributes which can be effectively transferred to create environments which evoke meaningful places.

Orientation toward environmental meaning versus environmental function is a relatively new line of inquiry in the field of environment and behavior (Rubinstein & Parmelee, 1992). Studies have indicated that environmental meaning results from individual experiences and factors such as personal and cultural filters or social constructs (Rapoport, 1982). It's inconceivable that researchers in environment-behavior studies will develop an objective predefined formula capable of externally grasping the meaning of *meaning*. Because as "self-defining and self-interpreting animals, we humans must enter our own webs of meaning to understand ourselves" (Cole, 1992). Still, architects should nurture a sensitivity to places in terms of their own experiences, and to realize the experiences of the recipients of their design. Moreover, environment-behavior studies should be a meeting place for the disciplines concerned with the question of environmental meaning in their attempt to develop logical, reliable, interpretable, and systematically predictive theories.

INTEGRATING ENVIRONMENT AND AGING INTO ARCHITECTURAL EDUCATION

This book is for those who are interested in teaching and learning about the field of environment and aging; for those who believe in choice and want to incorporate a sense of community into retirement life; for those who are seeking paths of innovations in design and management of facilities for eldercare; for those who pursue architecture as the meeting of behavioral and environmental disciplines and are working toward more humane retirement communities.

Existing patterns in the practice of architecture emphasize the packaging of architecture; architects are more interested in external and internal appearances of buildings than in their other meaningful aspects. Architectural practice is weakened by the tension between the view of architecture as art versus that of a science-based profession. Consequently, too often architects are concerned with images and styling rather than with the heart of things. History shows that ultimately only *understanding* permits effective change in desired and predictable ways. Valid practice is impossible without research and theoretical knowledge. This notion is crucial when one considers the field of gerontology, where the physical environment emphasizes independence and yet is responsive to the frailty of elderly people.

There is a need for research in the field of environment and aging that is not being met. Several factors may be responsible for the lack of activity in this important research domain in the past decade: (1) the relative standstill in federally assisted housing programs since 1980; (2) the relatively small trickle of new facilities for the elderly construction and the slowing of community development funds, both of which spurred the research of the 1970s (Parmelee & Lawton, 1990). But there seems to be another, more fundamental problem which affects research of environments and aging as well as the long-term care policies. Thomas Cole (1992) expressed it in his recent book:

> Our culture is not much interested in why we grow old, how we ought to grow old, or what it means to grow old. Like other aspects of our biological and social existence, aging has been brought under the dominion of scientific management, which is primarily interested in how we age in order to explain and control the aging process. (p. xx)

The equation of old age with illness has encouraged American society to think of aging as pathological or abnormal. The phenomenon and experience of aging was brought within the medical paradigm as an individual pathology to be treated and cured. Perhaps this is one of the reasons why the United States places a higher percentage of its elderly in medical model long-term care facilities than any other industrial nation in the world. Other cultures have believed that aging should be accepted, and that it should be, in part, a time of continued growth and yes, even preparation for death. Our culture seems increasingly to dispute that view, often preferring to think of aging as hardly more than another disease, to be fought and rejected. Suffice it to say, at this point, that research agendas are dominated by this approach. Similarly, the architecture of facilities for the elderly in the U.S. is embedded in the cultural history of aging, and is a physical reflection of the political and social policies toward the elderly in this country.

The development of the main theses that have been introduced here could be the basis for both academic and professional strengthening. Architects have always presented architecture as a responding art. They say: It needs a "client." And that device has frequently kept them from confronting moral or ethical issues. We disagree. We believe that architects and environmental designers should be in a steering position in the field of environment and aging. Steering requires people who see the entire universe of issues and possibilities and can balance competing demands for resources. Professional education should cultivate future leadership that will be able to contribute, through meaningful supportive environments, to the meaning and significance of later life.

REFERENCES

Cole, T. R. (1992). *The Journey of Life: A Cultural History of Aging in America*. Cambridge: Cambridge University Press.

Golant, S. M. (1992). *Housing America's Elderly: Many Possibilities/Few Choices*. Newbury Park, CA: Sage Publications.

Hillery, G. A. (1955). Definitions of community: Areas of agreement. *Rural Sociology*, 20, 111-123.

Lawton, M. P. (1987). Environment and the Need Satisfaction of the Aging. In L. L. Carstensen and B. A. Edelstein (Eds.) *Handbook of Clinical Gerontology*. New York: Pergamon Press.

Lawton, M. P., and Simon, B. (1968). The ecology of social relationships in housing for the elderly. *Gerontologist*, 8, 108-115.

Parmelee, P. A., and Lawton, M. P. (1990). The Design of Special Environments for the Aged. In J. E. Birren and W. Schaie (Eds.) *Handbook of the Psychology of Aging* (Third Edition). New York: Academic Press Inc.

Rapoport, A. (1982). *The Meaning of the Built Environment: A Nonverbal Communication Approach*. Beverly Hills, CA: Sage Publications.

Rubinstein, R. L., and Parmelee, P. A. (1992). Attachment to Place and the Representation of the Life Course by the Elderly. In I. Altman and S. M. Low (Eds.) *Place Attachment*. New York: Plenum Press.

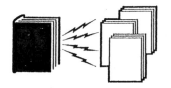

Haworth
DOCUMENT DELIVERY
SERVICE
and Local Photocopying Royalty Payment Form

This new service provides (a) a single-article order form for any article from a Haworth journal and (b) a convenient royalty payment form for local photocopying (not applicable to photocopies intended for resale).

- *Time Saving:* No running around from library to library to find a specific article.
- *Cost Effective:* All costs are kept down to a minimum.
- *Fast Delivery:* Choose from several options, including same-day FAX.
- *No Copyright Hassles:* You will be supplied by the original publisher.
- *Easy Payment:* Choose from several easy payment methods.

Open Accounts Welcome for . . .
- Library Interlibrary Loan Departments
- Library Network/Consortia Wishing to Provide Single-Article Services
- Indexing/Abstracting Services with Single Article Provision Services
- Document Provision Brokers and Freelance Information Service Providers

MAIL or *FAX* THIS ENTIRE ORDER FORM TO:

Attn: **Marianne Arnold**
Haworth Document Delivery Service
The Haworth Press, Inc.
10 Alice Street
Binghamton, NY 13904-1580

or **FAX:** (607) 722-1424
or **CALL:** 1-800-3-HAWORTH
(1-800-342-9678; 9am-5pm EST)

PLEASE SEND ME PHOTOCOPIES OF THE FOLLOWING SINGLE ARTICLES:
1) Journal Title: _____
   Vol/Issue/Year:_____ Starting & Ending Pages:_____
   Article Title:_____
   _____

2) Journal Title: _____
   Vol/Issue/Year:_____ Starting & Ending Pages:_____
   Article Title:_____
   _____

3) Journal Title: _____
   Vol/Issue/Year:_____ Starting & Ending Pages:_____
   Article Title:_____
   _____

4) Journal Title: _____
   Vol/Issue/Year:_____ Starting & Ending Pages:_____
   Article Title:_____
   _____

(See other side for Costs and Payment Information)

COSTS: Please figure your cost to order quality copies of an article.

1. Set-up charge per article: $8.00
   ($8.00 × number of separate articles) _____

2. Photocopying charge for each article:

   1-10 pages: $1.00 _____

   11-19 pages: $3.00 _____

   20-29 pages: $5.00 _____

   30+ pages: $2.00/10 pages _____

3. Flexicover (optional): $2.00/article _____

4. Postage & Handling: US: $1.00 for the first article/
   $.50 each additional article _____
   Federal Express: $25.00 _____
   Outside US: $2.00 for first article/
   $.50 each additional article _____

5. Same-day FAX service: $.35 per page _____

6. Local Photocopying Royalty Payment: should you wish to copy the article yourself. Not intended for photocopies made for resale. $1.50 per article per copy
   (i.e. 10 articles x $1.50 each = $15.00) _____

GRAND TOTAL: _____

METHOD OF PAYMENT: (please check one)

❑ Check enclosed   ❑ Please ship and bill. PO # _____
(sorry we can ship and bill to bookstores only! All others must pre-pay)

❑ Charge to my credit card: ❑ Visa; ❑ MasterCard; ❑ American Express;

Account Number: _____   Expiration date: _____

Signature: X _____   Name: _____

Institution: _____   Address: _____

City: _____   State: _____   Zip: _____

Phone Number: _____   FAX Number: _____

MAIL or *FAX* THIS ENTIRE ORDER FORM TO:

Attn: **Marianne Arnold**
Haworth Document Delivery Service
The Haworth Press, Inc.
10 Alice Street
Binghamton, NY 13904-1580

or FAX: (607) 722-1424
or CALL: 1-800-3-HAWORTH
(1-800-342-9678; 9am-5pm EST)